Preterm Premature Rupture of Membranes

Editors

EDWARD CHIEN
BRIAN M. MERCER

OBSTETRICS AND GYNECOLOGY CLINICS OF NORTH AMERICA

www.obgyn.theclinics.com

Consulting Editor
WILLIAM F. RAYBURN

December 2020 • Volume 47 • Number 4

ELSEVIER

1600 John F. Kennedy Boulevard • Suite 1800 • Philadelphia, Pennsylvania, 19103-2899

http://www.theclinics.com

OBSTETRICS AND GYNECOLOGY CLINICS OF NORTH AMERICA Volume 47, Number 4
December 2020 ISSN 0889-8545, ISBN-13: 978-0-323-77659-2

Editor: Kerry Holland
Developmental Editor: Kristen Helm

Obstetrics and Gynecology Clinics (ISSN 0889-8545) is published quarterly by Elsevier Inc., 360 Park Avenue South, New York, NY 10010-1710. Months of issue are March, June, September, and December. Periodicals postage paid at New York, NY, and additional mailing offices. Subscription price per year is $325.00 (US individuals), $719.00 (US institutions), $100.00 (US students), $404.00 (Canadian individuals), $908.00 (Canadian institutions), $100.00 (Canadian students), $459.00 (international individuals), $908.00 (international institutions), and $225.00 (international students). To receive student/resident rate, orders must be accompanied by name of affiliated institution, date of term, and the signature of program/residency coordinator on institution letterhead. Orders will be billed at individual rate until proof of status is received. Foreign air speed delivery is included in all *Clinics* subscription prices. All prices are subject to change without notice. POSTMASTER: Send address changes to *Obstetrics and Gynecology Clinics*, Elsevier Health Sciences Division, Subscription Customer Service, 3251 Riverport Lane, Maryland Heights, MO 63043. **Customer Service: Telephone: 1-800-654-2452 (U.S. and Canada); 314-447-8871 (outside U.S. and Canada). Fax: 314-447-8029. E-mail: journalscustomerservice-usa@elsevier.com (for print support); journalsonlinesupport-usa@elsevier. com (for online support).**

Reprints. For copies of 100 or more of articles in this publication, please contact the Commercial Reprints Department, Elsevier Inc., 360 Park Avenue South, New York, New York 10010-1710. Tel.: 212-633-3874; Fax: 212-633-3820; E-mail: reprints@elsevier.com.

Obstetrics and Gynecology Clinics of North America is also published in Spanish by McGraw-Hill Interamericana Editores S.A., P.O. Box 5-237, 06500, Mexico; in Portuguese by Reichmann and Affonso Editores, Rio de Janeiro, Brazil; and in Greek by Paschalidis Medical Publications, Athens, Greece.

Obstetrics and Gynecology Clinics of North America is covered in MEDLINE/PubMed (Index Medicus), Excerpta Medica, Current Concepts/Clinical Medicine, Science Citation Index, BIOSIS, CINAHL, and ISI/BIOMED.

Contributors

CONSULTING EDITOR

WILLIAM F. RAYBURN, MD, MBA
Adjunct Professor, Department of Obstetrics and Gynecology, College of Graduate Studies, Medical University of South Carolina, Charleston, South Carolina, USA; Emeritus Distinguished Professor, Department of Obstetrics and Gynecology, University of New Mexico School of Medicine, Albuquerque, New Mexico, USA

EDITORS

EDWARD CHIEN, MD, MBA
Chair of Obstetric and Gynecology Specialties, Cleveland Clinic, Women's Health Institute, Professor of Reproductive Biology, Case Western Reserve University, Cleveland, Ohio, USA

BRIAN M. MERCER, MD
Chair of Obstetrics and Gynecology, MetroHealth Medical Center, Professor of Reproductive Biology, Case Western Reserve University, Cleveland, Ohio, USA

AUTHORS

ASHLEY N. BATTARBEE, MD, MSCR
Assistant Professor, Department of Obstetrics and Gynecology, Center for Women's Reproductive Health, The University of Alabama at Birmingham, Birmingham, Alabama, USA

PHILLIP ROBERT BENNETT, BSc, PhD, MD, FRCOG, FMedSci
Director, Institute for Reproductive and Developmental Biology, Coordinating Director, March of Dimes European Prematurity Research Centre, Professor of Obstetrics and Gynaecology, Imperial College London, Kensington, London, United Kingdom; Honorary Consultant, Obstetrics and Gynaecology, Trust Director of Research for Woman's and Children's Health, Imperial Healthcare NHS Trust at Queen Charlottes Hospital

LILLIAN B. BOETTCHER, MD
Resident, Department of Obstetrics and Gynecology, University of Utah School of Medicine, Salt Lake City, Utah, USA

KERRI BRACKNEY, MD
Fellow, Maternal Fetal Medicine, Department of Obstetrics and Gynecology, Clinical Assistant Professor of Reproductive Biology, Case Western Reserve University, The MetroHealth System, Cleveland, Ohio, USA

RICHARD GAILON BROWN, BSc, MBBS, PhD, MRCOG
Honorary Clinical Research Fellow, March of Dimes European Prematurity Research Centre, Imperial College London, Kensington, London, United Kingdom

IRINA BURD, MD, PhD
Associate Professor, Department of Gynecology and Obstetrics, Division of Maternal-Fetal Medicine, Johns Hopkins School of Medicine, Baltimore, Maryland, USA

SUNEET P. CHAUHAN, MD, Hon DSc
Professor, Department of Obstetrics, Gynecology and Reproductive Sciences, McGovern Medical School, The University of Texas Health Science Center at Houston (UTHealth), Houston, Texas, USA

ERIN A.S. CLARK, MD
Associate Professor and Division Chief, Department of Obstetrics and Gynecology, University of Utah School of Medicine, Salt Lake City, Utah, USA

SARAH DOTTERS-KATZ, MD, MMHPE
Assistant Professor, Department of Obstetrics and Gynecology, Duke University, Duke University School of Medicine, Durham, North Carolina, USA

BRAXTON FORDE, MD
Clinical Associate, Division of Maternal-Fetal Medicine, Department of Obstetrics and Gynecology, University of Cincinnati College of Medicine, Cincinnati, Ohio, USA

LUKE A. GATTA, MD
Department of Obstetrics and Gynecology, Division of Maternal-Fetal Medicine, Duke University Hospital, Durham, North Carolina, USA

KELLY S. GIBSON, MD
Division Director, Maternal Fetal Medicine, Department of Obstetrics and Gynecology, Assistant Professor of Reproductive Biology, Case Western Reserve University, The MetroHealth System, Cleveland, Ohio, USA

MOUNIRA HABLI, MD
Division of Maternal-Fetal Medicine, Department of Obstetrics and Gynecology, Good Samaritan Hospital, Fetal Care Center of Cincinnati, Cincinnati Children's Hospital, Cincinnati, Ohio, USA

BRENNA L. HUGHES, MD, MSc
Department of Obstetrics and Gynecology, Division of Maternal-Fetal Medicine, Duke University Hospital, Durham, North Carolina, USA

EBONI O. JONES, MD
Physician, Department of Obstetrics and Gynecology, Lehigh Valley Health Network, Allentown, Pennsylvania, USA

DEEPAK KUMAR, MD
Professor, Department of Pediatrics, MetroHealth Medical Center, Case Western Reserve University, Cleveland, Ohio, USA

ZI-QI LIEW, MD
Physician, Department of Obstetrics and Gynecology, Lehigh Valley Health Network, Allentown, Pennsylvania, USA

DAVID ALAN MACINTYRE, BSc, PhD
Scientific Director, March of Dimes European Prematurity Research Centre, Reader in Reproductive Systems Medicine, Section Head, Pregnancy, Parturition and Prematurity, Imperial College London, Kensington, London, United Kingdom; Imperial College Faculty

of Medicine, Institute for Reproductive and Developmental Biology, London, United Kingdom

JOSEPH M. MANSOUR, PhD
Professor, Mechanical and Aerospace Engineering, Case Western Reserve University, Cleveland, Ohio, USA

HECTOR MENDEZ-FIGUEROA, MD
Associate Professor, Department of Obstetrics, Gynecology and Reproductive Sciences, McGovern Medical School, The University of Texas Health Science Center at Houston (UTHealth), Houston, Texas, USA

BRIAN M. MERCER, MD
Chair of Obstetrics and Gynecology, MetroHealth Medical Center, Professor of Reproductive Biology, Case Western Reserve University, Cleveland, Ohio, USA

JOHN J. MOORE, MD
Professor, Departments of Pediatrics, and Reproductive Biology, MetroHealth Medical Center, Case Western Reserve University, Cleveland, Ohio, USA

ROBERT M. MOORE, MS
Department of Pediatrics, MetroHealth Medical Center, Case Western Reserve University, Cleveland, Ohio, USA

ORION A. RUST, MD
Physician, Department of Obstetrics and Gynecology, Lehigh Valley Health Network, Allentown, Pennsylvania, USA

ANGELA K. SHADDEAU, MD, MS
Clinical Fellow, Department of Gynecology and Obstetrics, Division of Maternal-Fetal Medicine, Johns Hopkins School of Medicine, Baltimore, Maryland, USA

Contents

There is an association between vaginal microbiota dysbiosis and preterm
premature rupture of membranes (PPROM). In PPROM, reduced *Lactobacillus* spp abundance is linked to the emergence of high-risk vaginal microbiota, close to the time of membrane rupture. Although PPROM itself can
change vaginal microbial composition, antibiotic therapy profoundly effects community structure. Erythromycin may have a beneficial effect in
women deplete in *Lactobacillus* spp but damages a healthy microbiome
by targeting *Lactobacillus* spp Increased rates of chorioamnionitis and
early-onset neonatal sepsis are associated with vaginal microbiota dysbiosis close to the time of delivery.

Using a novel in vitro model system combining biochemical/histologic with
bioengineering approaches has provided significant insights into the physiology of fetal membrane weakening and rupture along with potential
mechanistic reasons for lack of efficacy of currently clinically used agents
to prevent preterm premature rupture of the membranes (PPROM) and
preterm births. Likewise, the model has also facilitated screening of agents
with potential for preventing PPROM and preterm birth.

A short cervix in the second trimester is a significant risk factor for spontaneous preterm birth, preterm prelabor rupture of membranes, and subsequent adverse perinatal outcome. The pathophysiology is complex
and multifactorial with inflammatory and/or infectious processes often
involved. Biomarkers have been developed in an effort to predict preterm
birth with varying degrees of success. The treatment options of cerclage,
progesterone, pessary, and combination therapy are reviewed.
Evidence-based protocols are summarized for singleton and multiple
gestation.

Trials evaluating tocolytic use in preterm premature rupture of membranes (PPROM) have been small and lacked adequate power to evaluate uncommon outcomes. There still is much controversy on the benefit, length of use, route, and drug of choice among clinicians treating patients with PPROM. Most professional medical societies would propose to consider the use of tocolytics for 48 hours to allow for corticosteroid administration or to allow for maternal transfer to a higher level of care. Longer treatment regimens may lead to adverse maternal and perinatal outcomes. Insufficient data are available to make stronger and more definitive recommendations.

Antenatal corticosteroids are important interventions to prevent neonatal morbidity and mortality associated with preterm birth. Administering intramuscular betamethasone or dexamethasone before preterm birth reduces risks of respiratory distress syndrome, intraventricular hemorrhage, necrotizing enterocolitis, and death. These same benefits are seen among women with preterm prelabor rupture of membranes (PPROM) without any proven increased risk of neonatal or maternal infection. Although future studies are needed to elucidate effects of antenatal corticosteroids at less than 23 weeks' gestation and a rescue course at later gestational ages after PPROM, a single course of antenatal corticosteroids is vital to optimizing neonatal outcomes after PPROM.

For many years, providers have been using antibiotics to prevent infection in women who present with preterm prelabor rupture of membranes (PPROM). Given the polymicrobial nature of intra-amniotic infection, the recommended regimen includes a 7-day course of ampicillin and erythromycin, although many substitute of azithromycin. This regimen is used from viability to 34 weeks, independent of the number of fetuses present. Meta-analyses have shown that antibiotics for this indication are associated with lower rates of maternal and fetal infection, as well as longer pregnancy latency. Thus, latency antibiotics are recommended for all women with PPROM through 34 weeks of gestation.

Treatment of viral infections is geared toward ameliorating maternal symptoms and minimizing perinatal transmission. Multidisciplinary teams often are required to manage sequelae due to viral diseases in patients with preterm premature rupture of membranes (PPROM). Although data are scarce regarding the antepartum management of common viruses in PPROM, essential principles may be extrapolated from national guidelines and studies in gravid patients. The well-established risks of prematurity are weighed against the often unclear risks of vertical transmission.

Preterm prelabor rupture of membranes is a complication of pregnancy with significant associated maternal and fetal risks. Expectant management of this complication requires inpatient admission with close monitoring of maternal and fetal status until delivery. Close antepartum monitoring ensures rapid intervention if indicated, allowing for best possible maternal and neonatal outcomes.

Special Topics

Periviable deliveries (less than 26 weeks) are a small percentage of deliveries but account for a disproportionately high number of long-term morbidities. Few studies describe interventions and outcomes for periviable preterm premature rupture of membranes (PPROM). The available reports may include only those neonates who received resuscitation, making interpretation and application difficult. Counseling should consider the impact of oligohydramnios on fetal lung development. This article discusses standard and experimental interventions that may offer neonatal benefit. Antenatal corticosteroids, antibiotics, and magnesium sulfate may improve outcomes but data to support an improvement in outcome are limited. Studies specifically evaluating these interventions are needed.

Two unique aspects of antenatal care occur in the setting of fetal surgery and multiple gestations. As fetal interventions increase, so do the number of cases of iatrogenic preterm prelabor rupture of membranes (PPROM). Because of the amniotic sac's inability to heal, the risk of PPROM after surgery is directly correlated with the number of interventions, the size of the defect, and the surgery performed. Higher order gestations also carry an increased risk of PPROM. This paper reviews the risks and management of PPROM in the setting of the various prenatal interventions as well as in the setting of multiple gestations.

Preterm premature rupture of membranes (PPROM) is almost uniformly associated with preterm birth and thus sequelae of prematurity explain many of the complications associated with this condition. However, the unique inflammatory environment and oligohydramnios associated with PPROM may impart unique neonatal and childhood morbidity compared with other preterm birth pathways.

OBSTETRICS AND GYNECOLOGY CLINICS

SERIES OF RELATED INTEREST

Clinics in Perinatology
www.perinatology.theclinics.com
Pediatric Clinics of North America
www.pediatrics.theclinics.com

THE CLINICS ARE AVAILABLE ONLINE!
Access your subscription at:
www.theclinics.com

Foreword

Premature Rupture of Membranes: The Most Common Factor Leading to Preterm Birth

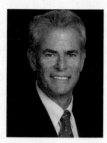

William F. Rayburn, MD, MBA
Consulting Editor

Preterm premature rupture of the membranes (PPROM) before 37 weeks, 0 days is responsible for or associated with one in every 3 preterm births and is the most commonly identified factor associated with preterm birth. This issue of *Obstetrics and Gynecology Clinics of North America*, capably coedited by Edward Chien, MD, MBA and Brian M. Mercer, MD, from Case Western Reserve University, addresses problems resulting from premature rupture of the membranes that contribute to significant morbidity and mortality. The articles are nicely divided into 3 important sections: prediction and prevention, interventions, and special topics.

The pathogenesis of PPROM is incompletely understood. Several events (eg, altered vaginal microbiome, inflammation, membrane weakening, short cervix, and bleeding) have been implicated, which initiates a series of biochemical changes culminating in membrane rupture. The most common risk factors include a history of PPROM, genital tract infection, and cigarette smoking. The classic presentation is a sudden "gush" or wetness of clear or pale-yellow fluid. A sterile speculum examination allows for direct observation of cervical dilation and the fluid leaking from the cervical internal orifice and pooling in the vaginal vault, either spontaneously or after pushing on her fundus, Valsalva maneuver, or coughing.

Although still commonly used, obtaining vaginal fluid for nitrazine or fern tests is being replaced by commercial tests that have fewer false positive and higher positive predictive values. Commercial tests are available to test the fluid at the point of care to detect placental alpha-macroglobulin, placental protein 12, and alpha-fetoprotein. Their routine use is questioned, however. Ultrasonography is often used as an adjunct to confirm oligohydramnios when tests demonstrate discrepancies in results.

Obstet Gynecol Clin N Am 47 (2020) xi–xii
https://doi.org/10.1016/j.ogc.2020.09.003
0889-8545/20/© 2020 Published by Elsevier Inc.

obgyn.theclinics.com

Management decisions about PPROM are among the most controversial in perinatal medicine. Any intervention is based upon several factors, which are assessed upon presentation: gestational age, any maternal/fetal infection, any labor, fetal presentation, fetal heart rate and uterine activity recordings, expectation of fetal lung maturity, cervical status on visual inspection, and level of neonatal care. Points of contention discussed in this issue include expectant management versus intervention, use of tocolytics, duration of antibiotic administration, timing of antenatal corticosteroids, and methods of testing for maternal/fetal infection.

Perhaps the most important management decision is timing of preterm delivery. This issue highlights components of expectant management: monitoring fetal well-being, administering antenatal corticosteroids, screening for infections including group B streptococcus, and administering a 7-day course of prophylactic antibiotics using a drug regimen (with or without a penicillin allergy that is low or high risk for anaphylaxis). As mentioned in the issue, unproven interventions include supplemental progesterone, tissue sealants (eg, fibrin glue, or gelatin sponge), and amnioinfusion. Prompt delivery is appropriate in the presence of suspected intrauterine infection, nonreassuring fetal testing, or placental abruption. Discussions about route of delivery and magnesium sulfate for neuroprotection are then undertaken.

Special considerations are reviewed in this issue. Separate articles include topics about pregnancies with periviable PPROM, recent fetal surgery, and neonatal and childhood outcomes following PPROM. Morbidity and mortality are primarily related to preterm birth, coexisting fetal structural abnormalities, residual oligohydramnios, and coexisting chorioamnionitis. Other areas of special interest in this issue include the following topics: indications for tocolysis; hospitalization versus home care; concurrent viral infection; presence of a cerclage; meconium-stained fluid; twin gestations; and management of future pregnancies. Use of prophylactic progesterone supplementation, sonographic measurement of cervical length, and placement of a cerclage before 24 weeks are discussed to reduce a recurrent PROM in any subsequent gestation.

Topics in this issue address some of the most common interventions, which are either evidence-based or emerging. The clarity of the articles prepared by the experienced authors, with edits from Dr Chien and Dr Mercer, activates our attention to all issues of PPROM. Practical information provided herein will aid in the development and implementation of new guidelines and treatment options as this twenty-first century progresses.

William F. Rayburn, MD, MBA
Department of Obstetrics and Gynecology
University of New Mexico School of Medicine
MSC 10 5580, 1 University of New Mexico
Albuquerque, NM 87131-0001, USA

E-mail address:
wrayburnmd@gmail.com

Preface

Preterm Premature Rupture of the Membranes in the Twenty-First Century

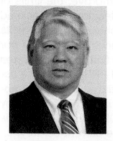 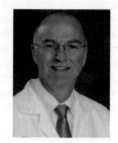

Edward Chien, MD, MBA   Brian M. Mercer, MD
Editors

Preterm rupture of the membranes continues to vex the obstetric community in the twenty-first century. This is one of the most frequent problems seen by the obstetric community that continues to contribute to significant morbidity and mortality, making it an important topic to be addressed in this issue of *Obstetrics and Gynecology Clinics of North America*. Within this issue, topics are divided into 3 sections: Prediction and Prevention, Interventions, and Special Topics.

The first section, Prediction and Prevention, provides background information related to the vaginal microbiome and fetal membrane biology and biomechanics. The vaginal flora is a dynamic environment that plays both a protective and a pathologic role in health and disease. Since the successful completion of the Human Genome Project, many other genomes have been determined. As we learn more about microbiomes, it is clear that they contribute to both health and disease. The article on the vaginal microbiome addresses current understanding of its role in outcomes related to preterm premature rupture of the membranes (PPROM). Our knowledge of the biomechanics of the fetal membrane continues to advance. The focus of our understanding has moved from compositional biology to biomechanics and molecular biology. This article provides food for thought and identifies potential therapeutic targets. This section ends by addressing the role of the cervix in PPROM. The shortening of the cervix is one of the few markers that have been recognized that identify individuals at risk for PPROM. This article addresses the role of cervical length along with the potential benefit of cervical cerclage.

The second section, Interventions, covers the literature around the use of tocolytics, antibiotics, corticosteroids, and antenatal monitoring. The vast majority of the research at the end of the twentieth century focused on these interventions. These interventions,

Obstet Gynecol Clin N Am 47 (2020) xiii–xiv
https://doi.org/10.1016/j.ogc.2020.09.002
0889-8545/20/© 2020 Published by Elsevier Inc.

along with the advances in neonatal medicine, have brought about a marked improvement in outcomes, giving parents and families much greater hope than at the beginning of that century. The twentieth century began with the Spanish flu pandemic in 1918, while this publication comes out in the midst of the SARS-CoV-2/COVID-19 pandemic. Although it is still too early to understand how COVID-19 will impact pregnancy and long-term outcomes, viral illnesses can impact the management of PPROM. We felt it was important for us to address some of these issues for relatively common viruses that impact pregnancy in the twenty-first century.

The final section addresses topics that are emerging or are continuing to emerge during the twenty-first century. As neonatal care continues to improve, the limits of viability continue to be a moving target. It seems that each decade is associated with a new gestational definition for viability. As this definition changes, the benefits of interventions are less clear. This article discusses the evidence for some of our common interventions in the periviable period. This century has finally demonstrated benefits of fetal interventions in utero, which has led to cases of PPROM that we assume are related to the disruption of the fetal membranes associated with these procedures. Are the management and outcomes different in this situation? The article by Forde and Habli discusses the impact of fetal surgery on PPROM. Finally, this issue addresses the marked improvement In neonatal outcomes in the current century.

We hope that this issue of *Obstetrics and Gynecology Clinics of North America* inspires new innovations and improves outcomes as this century progresses. It would be great to know what the care will be like at the end of the century.

Edward Chien, MD, MBA
Cleveland Clinic
Women's Health Institute
9500 Euclid Avenue, A81
Cleveland, OH 44195, USA

Brian M. Mercer, MD
MetroHealth Medical Center
2500 Metrohealth Drive
Cleveland, OH 44109, USA

E-mail addresses:
chiene@ccf.org (E. Chien)
bmercer@metrohealth.org (B.M. Mercer)

PREDICTION AND PREVENTION

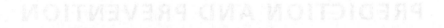

Vaginal Microbiome in Preterm Rupture of Membranes

Phillip Robert Bennett, BSc, PhD, MD, FRCOG, FMedSci[a,b,c],
Richard Gailon Brown, BSc, MBBS, PhD, MRCOG[a,c],
David Alan MacIntyre, BSc, PhD[a,b,*]

KEYWORDS

• Vaginal microbiome • PPROM • Membranes • Preterm birth • Inflammation

KEY POINTS

• There is an association between reduced *Lactobacillus* spp relative abundance and increased bacterial diversity in the maternal vaginal microbiota and risk of preterm premature rupture of membranes (PPROM).

• High-risk vaginal microbiota linked to PPROM are observed closer to the time of membrane rupture, although dominance of the vaginal microbiota by non-*Lactobacillus* spp at any gestational age increases risk.

• The event of PPROM itself may change vaginal microbiota structure in some women; however, antibiotic therapy appears to have a more significant effect and associates with increased rates of dysbiosis.

• Depletion of *Lactobacillus* spp within the vagina and the emergence of pathogenic microbiota close to delivery associate with chorioamnionitis and early-onset neonatal sepsis, which are risk factors for cerebral palsy.

• Women who have had excisional cervical surgery are at high risk of PPROM through mechanical factors and will do well with cervical cerclage if they have a short cervix, although choice of suture material may affect outcomes.

INTRODUCTION

Preterm birth (PTB) is one of the largest challenges facing obstetrics in the modern era. It is the leading cause of childhood mortality, is associated with 80% of all neonatal

[a] Institute for Reproductive and Developmental Biology, Faculty of Medicine, Imperial College London W12 0NN, UK; [b] March of Dimes European Prematurity Research Centre, Imperial College London W12 0NN, UK; [c] Imperial Healthcare NHS Trust at Queen Charlotte's Hospital, London, UK
* Corresponding author. Institute for Reproductive and Developmental Biology, Faculty of Medicine, Imperial College London, Hammersmith Hospital Campus, Du Cane Road, London W12 0NN, UK.
E-mail address: d.macintyre@imperial.ac.uk

Obstet Gynecol Clin N Am 47 (2020) 503–521
https://doi.org/10.1016/j.ogc.2020.08.001
0889-8545/20/© 2020 Elsevier Inc. All rights reserved.
obgyn.theclinics.com

morbidity,[1] and results in unparalleled financial and emotional cost to families and society. Preterm premature rupture of membranes (PPROM) is a major feature of the PTB syndrome, preceding 30% to 40% of cases.[2] Many of the causes are incompletely understood, and the incidence continues to increase on a global scale.[3] As with preterm labor, more generally, PPROM can be considered to be a syndrome with multiple underlying causes. A wide range of epidemiologic and clinical factors has been associated with PPROM. It is more common in multifetal pregnancy, and in pregnancies complicated by polyhydramnios, suggesting a role for mechanical forces. It has also been linked to cigarette smoking, substance abuse, and poor nutritional status. However, the pathogenesis of membrane rupture and subsequent maternal and neonatal morbidities is strongly associated with infection.[4,5] PPROM has a higher association with infection and inflammation than does preterm delivery without prior PPROM and is associated with a significantly lower gestational age and birth weight and higher rates of chorioamnionitis, urinary tract infection, endometritis, and postpartum bacteremia.[6-8]

Bacterial vaginosis,[9,10] aerobic vaginitis,[11] and colonization of the lower reproductive tract with pathogens, including trichomoniasis, gonorrhea, and chlamydia,[11] have been associated with second-trimester miscarriage, PPROM, and PTB.[12] It has been hypothesized that colonization of the vagina with pathogenic bacteria activates the innate immune system of the vagina, cervix, fetal membranes, and decidua,[2,13] driving an inflammatory cascade[14-17] that leads to oxidative stress, immune cell influx, upregulation of prostaglandins and metalloproteinases, downregulation of proteases inhibitors, and induction of apoptosis, culminating in cervical remodeling and disruption of membrane architecture resulting in PPROM.[13,18,19] Following PPROM, the uterine cavity, placenta, and fetus are exposed to vaginal microbiota, increasing the risk of chorioamnionitis, funisitis, and colonization of the neonate, which associates with poor maternal and neonatal outcomes.[20-26] Antibiotic treatment does not consistently reduce the rate of PPROM or PTB[27] or improve outcomes, suggesting suboptimal treatment strategies or inaccurate identification of the underlying cause.

Menon and colleagues[28] have shown that fetal leukocyte telomere length reduces in association with normal term labor. Telomere length serves as a surrogate for fetal stress and placental membrane senescence and as a marker for oxidative stress. Telomere length is reduced in PPROM compared with PTB without prior PPROM but is similar to term births, suggesting that PPROM represents a placental membrane disease mediated by oxidative stress-induced senescence. The differences in fetal leukocyte telomere length between cases of PPROM and PTB suggest distinct pathophysiologic processes that differentiate these outcomes. A range of factors, including cigarette smoking, substance abuse, nutritional deficiencies, and infection or inflammation, each of which is a recognized risk for PPROM, can lead to imbalances in the redox status resulting in oxidative stress. Mechanical stress may also activate inflammatory mediators via activation of the NFκB and AP-1 transcription factor systems within the fetal membranes,[29] providing an attractive integrated hypothesis for a final common pathway to membrane rupture.

DNA SEQUENCING-BASED INTERROGATION OF THE MICROBIOME

Bacteria were identified as determinants of health and disease in the late nineteenth century. Research throughout the twentieth century laid the foundation of the current understanding of microbiology but was limited by culture-dependent methodologies. In the early twenty-first century, advances in DNA sequencing techniques provided the technology to comprehensively and rapidly characterize polymicrobial communities.[30]

The term "microbiome" is often used interchangeably with "microbiota" to mean the assemblage of microorganisms present in a defined environment. More correctly, however, the "microbiome" refers to the entire habitat, including the microorganisms, their genomes, and the surrounding environmental conditions.[31] A further issue in relation to the term "microbiome" is that some investigators consider that it should only be applied to microbial communities that have some biological or physiologic function beyond its own simple existence. For example, the human gut microbiome has a high microbial biomass and plays a wide range of essential physiologic functions in addition to nutrient absorption of vitamins, amino acids, and short-chain fatty acids. These functions include enzyme synthesis, maintenance of mucosal integrity, immunomodulation, and protection against pathogens.[32] The human vaginal microbiome has a moderately high microbial biomass and plays important roles in protecting the vagina from overgrowth of pathobionts and pathogens, and therefore reducing the risk of ascending pelvic inflammatory disease or chorioamnionitis.[33] These 2 "microbiomes" clearly have essential physiologic functions. The human placenta, on the other hand, may in some cases harbor small numbers of microorganisms, but the structure of the "microbiome" is not consistent, and convincing evidence for an essential physiologic role for bacteria within the placenta in normal pregnancy is lacking.[34,35]

The metagenome, which describes the collection of genomes and genes from the members of a microbiota, can be obtained through shotgun sequencing of DNA by assembly, mapping to a reference database, and annotation. Metagenomic analyses have the advantages of providing information about the genetics of all the constituents of the habitat and thus can be used to infer potential function of a community in addition to its compositional structure. However, metagenomics has a higher economic and computational cost and can be problematic to apply to low bacterial biomass human samples (eg, placenta) where most sequenced DNA is of host origin. Sequencing of large amounts of host DNA can be circumvented by metataxonomics, which relies on the amplification and sequencing of taxonomic marker genes, most commonly the bacterial 16S ribosomal RNA gene. The 16S ribosomal gene is composed of highly conserved regions and 9 "hypervariable" regions (V1–V9). The conserved regions permit binding of polymerase chain reaction primers for amplification, whereas the variable regions are diverse and distinctive, enabling classification of bacterial taxonomy to species and in some cases strain level.[36] However, metataxonomics approaches are prone to bias because of choice of amplification region, primer design, and the pipeline used for analysis and are unable to robustly inform on bacterial function or metabolism. Currently, most studies examining the reproductive tract microbiota, particularly in pregnancy, have used metataxonomics.

THE PREGNANCY VAGINAL MICROBIOME

There is now substantial evidence linking the structure of the vaginal microbiota with PPROM and PTB. Recent studies that have used molecular-based approaches to investigate the vaginal microbiota have produced findings that are largely consistent with earlier culture-dependent methods that identified *Lactobacillus* spp as the predominant vaginal commensal in pregnancy. However, the advent of next-generation sequencing has enabled more detailed characterization of the complexity and dynamics of the vaginal microbiota, and many of the observations identified by culture dependent techniques are being revisited.

The microbiota of the female reproductive tract fluctuates throughout a woman's lifespan and in response to circulating hormone levels. The microbiome is first established shortly after birth when the neonate is exposed to maternal microbiota.[37] Before menarche, the vaginal microbiome is diverse and consists of aerobic, anaerobic, and enteric bacteria.[38] As menarche approaches, rising estrogen levels promote proliferation of vaginal epithelial cells and glycogen deposition. The thickened vaginal epithelium produces lactic acid,[39] causing a decrease in pH that favors colonization by acidophilic bacteria, such as *Lactobacillus* spp. Lactobacilli metabolize the rich glycogen stores producing lactate isomers that further reduce the pH of the vaginal mucosa. Few other microorganisms are able to tolerate these conditions, and *Lactobacillus* spp emerge as the dominant commensal in most individuals.[40] Dominance of the vaginal niche is also achieved by *Lactobacillus* spp through competitive exclusion and the production of compounds, such as bacteriocins[41] and biosurfactants.[42] The environment created provides the host protection against pathogenic colonization associated with bacterial vaginosis,[43,44] pelvic inflammatory disease,[45] candidiasis,[46] sexually transmitted infections, human immunodeficiency virus, herpes simplex virus-2, and carcinogenic human papilloma virus.[47]

In most women, *Lactobacillus* spp dominance persists throughout the reproductive years.[48] The first metataxonomic analysis of the microbiota of nonpregnant, asymptomatic women, by Ravel and colleagues,[48] used hierarchical clustering methods to describe 5 distinct community state types (CST); four of these state types: CST I (*Lactobacillus crispatus*), CST II (*Lactobacillus gasseri*), CST III (*Lactobacillus iners*), and CST V (*Lactobacillus jensenii*), are *Lactobacillus* spp dominant; the fifth, CST IV, is characterized by a *Lactobacillus* spp–depleted polymicrobial community enriched with *Gardnerella vaginalis*, *Atopobium vaginae*, *Megasphaera*, *Peptoniphilus*, *Sneathia*, *Finegoldia*, *Prevotella*, *Dialister*, and *Mobiluncus* spp. CST IV was thus compositionally similar to bacterial vaginosis and was predominately observed in black and Hispanic women compared with women of Asian and white ethnicity. Further studies indicate that ethnic[49] and geographic[50,51] variation in vaginal microbiota is not completely explained by socioeconomic, dietary, sexual, or personal hygiene factors[49] and highlights the potential genetic component to microbiome acquisition.

During pregnancy, placental metabolism leads to a marked increase in circulating estrogen concentrations[52] with a consequent reduction in vaginal bacterial diversity and promotion of *Lactobacillus* spp dominance.[50,51,53] Following delivery, maternal estrogen levels decrease almost 1000-fold,[52] and passage of lochia dramatically alters the vaginal environment resulting in decreased *Lactobacillus* spp and a shift toward a *Lactobacillus* spp–depleted community structure that can persist for up to 1 year postpartum.[54]

THE VAGINAL MICROBIOTA AND PRETERM BIRTH

Early reports examining the relationship between vaginal microbiota composition and PTB using culture-independent methods reported inconsistent results that were likely reflective of geographic and ethnic variation of study populations, limited cohort sizes and statistical power, and a heterogeneous mix of PTB causes, many of which were late PTBs (36–37 weeks of gestation) and thus less likely to be of an infectious cause.[54–59] However, consideration of more recent studies that have focused on larger patient populations and/or careful characterization of PTB cause suggests the emergence of broadly consistent concepts.[59–70] Investigations in Europe[67,69,70] and Northern America[63,65,66,68] on predominantly Caucasian populations have consistently reported positive associations between increased vaginal microbial diversity and risk of PTB with many of these studies identifying *G vaginalis*, *Sneathia* spp, *Prevotella* spp, and *Mollicutes* spp as microbial markers of risk.[61–66,68] Conversely, studies in the United States performed in black women have reported decreased vaginal diversity as a risk factor[59,71] or have not shown any correlation between the vaginal microbiome and preterm risk.[58]

Although the aforementioned studies have used a variety of sequencing platforms and have targeted different regions of the hypervariable 16S rRNA gene for amplification, many of them have linked L crispatus dominance of the vaginal microbiota with healthy term pregnancy. In 2017, the authors reported in a cohort of 161 women, of whom 34 ultimately delivered preterm, that L crispatus dominance of the vaginal microbiome at 16 weeks of pregnancy appeared to confer protection against subsequent PTB. Various cross-sectionally and longitudinally sampled cohorts have since confirmed this observation and highlighted a relationship between Lactobacillus spp dominance and protection against PTB.[61,62,64,68]

VAGINAL MICROBIOTA AND THE SUBSEQUENT RISK OF PRETERM PREMATURE RUPTURE OF MEMBRANES

Only a limited number of studies have specifically examined the relationship between the vaginal microbiota and the subsequent risk of PPROM. In 2 recent publications, the authors examined the composition of vaginal microbiota during pregnancy before membrane rupture.[62,72] In the first of these, 250 women, predefined at high risk for PTB, were enrolled in a prospective cohort study in which they were sampled at 4 time points in pregnancy between 8 and 36 weeks.[62] A second cohort of 87 women were recruited upon presentation, after PPROM had occurred. Of the 250 women in the prospective series, 38 delivered preterm of whom 15 experienced PPROM. Although vaginal microbial communities isolated from the control women were, as expected, characterized by low diversity and Lactobacillus spp dominance, nearly half of the women sampled antenatally who subsequently experienced PPROM had a higher proportion intermediate or low Lactobacillus spp dominance and high diversity. These differences remained when analyses were adjusted for maternal age, ethnicity, body mass index, smoking status, and antenatal treatment interventions. This study thereby underscored the high rate of vaginal dysbiosis immediately before PPROM and suggested at least 2 "phenotypes" of PPROM, one linked to vaginal dysbiosis and the other not.

To examine the evolution of the vaginal microbiota during pregnancy before PPROM in more detail, the authors then undertook a study of 1500 women prospectively sampled from the first trimester of pregnancy, to identify 60 women who subsequently experienced PPROM.[72] Reduced Lactobacillus spp abundance and high diversity were observed in a quarter of women before PPROM, but in only 3% of women who delivered at term. PPROM was associated with instability of bacterial community structure during pregnancy and a shift toward higher diversity, predominately occurring during the second trimester. This study also suggested an effect of ethnicity on the vaginal microbiota, although numbers were insufficient for definitive conclusions. In women with subsequent PPROM, there was an increase in the number of women with a Lactobacillus spp–depleted vaginal microbiome across all ethnicities, with the greatest increase of Lactobacillus spp–depleted communities in black women. Although in general PPROM was associated with a shift toward higher diversity occurring during the second trimester, vaginal bacterial community dominated by any species other than Lactobacillus was associated with subsequent PPROM at all gestational time windows, including during the first trimester. In separate analyses of the relationship between vaginal microbiota and first-trimester miscarriage in the same cohort, the authors found that miscarriage also associates with a Lactobacillus spp–depleted vaginal microbiome,[73] and that women who have a threatened miscarriage in the first trimester had a subsequent 2-fold increased risk of PTB and 3-fold increased risk of PPROM.[74] These data suggest a link between miscarriage and PPROM associated with the early pregnancy microbiome.

VAGINAL MICROBIOTA AT THE TIME OF PRETERM PREMATURE RUPTURE OF MEMBRANES

A 2015 Czech study sampled 61 women at a single time point just after PPROM, before the administration of antibiotics. Samples were obtained from both the cervix and amniotic fluid, and the microbiome of each was analyzed in combination with cytokine levels and placental histology. Hierarchical clustering analysis demonstrated that the microbiome from cervical samples was categorized into 4 groups, which were consistent with the previously described CSTs, CST I (*L crispatus*), CST III (*L iners*) CST IVA (nonlactobacillus), and CST IVB (*G vaginalis/Sneathia* spp).[75] The lack of detection of other CSTs may represent a regional or ethnic difference, but more likely is a feature of the sample size. CST IVA and B were associated with higher cytokine levels and rates of microbial invasion of the amniotic cavity (MIAC). In contrast, CST I was associated with the lowest levels of inflammation and MIAC. In this study, 70% of PPROM pregnancies were complicated by histologic chorioamnionitis, which was subdivided into 2 subgroups: infectious and noninfectious, based on the presence or absence of MIAC. The combination of MIAC and histologic chorioamnionitis was found to represent a subgroup of PPROM with the strongest fetal inflammatory response. Low rates of MIAC with histologic chorioamnionitis were found in both of the *Lactobacillus* dominated CSTs, while high rates were seen in each of the non-*Lactobacillus* dominated CSTs.

The "PPROM study group" in Canada enrolled 36 women after PPROM, 19 of whom were sampled in series and reported increased vaginal microbial diversity with *Mycoplasma* and *Prevotella* spp being identified in all samples. They also showed that the microbiome during the latency period was unstable, fluctuating between a variety of non-*Lactobacillus* spp; however, there were no associations identified between microbiome profiles latency and neonatal outcome.[76]

In the earlier mentioned study of 87 women who were recruited on presentation after PPROM had occurred,[62] there were 39 cases of PPROM from whom vaginal swabs were taken before any antibiotic therapy had been started. Of these, nearly half had a vaginal microbiota characterized by intermediate or low *Lactobacillus* spp dominance and high diversity. These proportions were essentially identical to the proportions seen in women sampled close to, but before PPROM. However, in individual cases whereby samples were obtained both before and after PPROM, about half of those with *Lactobacillus* spp dominance before PPROM became dysbiotic after rupture (**Fig. 1**). These data suggest that in some cases the event of PPROM itself does significantly affect microbiome structure, which may be due to the alkalinity and presence of antimicrobial peptides in amniotic fluid.[77] However, PPROM was also associated with a reduction in overall bacterial load, which may represent washing out of bacteria in response to the rupture event. Taken together, the data from these studies again support the hypothesis that PPROM may be divisible into at least 2 broad phenotypes, an infection-mediated phenotype whereby the vaginal microbiota play an important etiologic role and a noninfectious phenotype driven by other factors.

EFFECTS OF ANTIBIOTICS ON THE VAGINAL MICROBIOTA AT THE TIME OF PRETERM PREMATURE RUPTURE OF MEMBRANES

The clinical management of PPROM generally involves a careful but difficult balance between prolongation of pregnancy to enable fetal maturation, and risk of infection

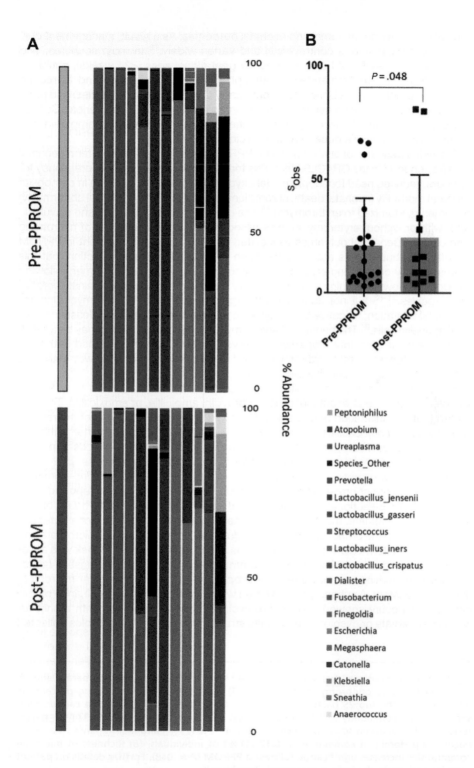

and subsequent poor maternal and neonatal outcomes. As a result, management during this latency period is controversial and varies widely.[78] In most countries, and particularly where PPROM occurs at earlier gestational ages (<34 weeks), antibiotic therapy is usually recommended to attempt to prolong pregnancy and to reduce neonatal morbidity. In the United Kingdom, many Commonwealth countries, and parts of Europe, there is widespread use of erythromycin in PPROM. The American College of Obstetricians and Gynecologists guidelines suggest a regimen of ampicillin and erythromycin or a single dose of azithromycin.

The widespread use of erythromycin for PPROM is based on the short-term neonatal benefits reported in the ORACLE I trial. This trial reported prolongation of pregnancy for 48 hours, reduced need for supplemental oxygen and a reduction (2.2%) in composite neonatal morbidity (neonatal death, chronic lung disease, or major cerebral abnormality) in women randomized to erythromycin.[79] The combination of amoxicillin and clavulanic acid, with or without erythromycin, was associated with increased risk of necrotizing enterocolitis. Beneficial outcomes associated with erythromycin treatment in PPROM are often attributed to its assumed inhibition of ascending vaginal infection, but this seems unlikely considering erythromycin concentration in the vaginal lumen following oral dosing is low,[80] reaching a mean inhibitory concentration effective against Lactobacillus species,[81–83] but not against most vaginal pathogens.[81] Erythromycin inhibits neutrophil migration, oxidative burst, cytokine, and metalloproteinase release in bronchial epithelial cells.[84] The benefits of erythromycin in the ORACLE I trial may be a result of these anti-inflammatory properties. However, in vitro studies performed in the authors' laboratory show that erythromycin fails to inhibit inflammatory pathway activation in amnion and vaginal epithelial cells (**Fig. 2**).

In a study by Baldwin and colleagues,[86] a proportion of the cohort (n = 9) was sampled before and after antibiotics (azithromycin, ampicillin, or amoxicillin). They reported that administration of these antibiotics did not significantly impact the relative abundance of Lactobacillus, Prevotella, or Peptoniphilus during or after antibiotic exposure, yet Weeksella, Lachnospira, Achromobacter, and Pediococcus spp were significantly decreased and Peptostreptococcus and Tissierellaceae ph2 were increased. It is worth noting that most of these cases had non-Lactobacillus–dominant vaginal microbiota at presentation. In contrast, the authors previously reported in an analysis of cross-sectional samples taken after PPROM following 48 hours of oral erythromycin treatment, that there was a general shift toward dysbiosis characterized by a reduction in the proportion of Lactobacillus spp–dominant vaginal microbiota and an increase in intermediate-type communities.[62] Treatment beyond 1 week was associated with a reduction of intermediate communities and a modest increase in Lactobacillus spp dominance. However, the proportion of dysbiotic vaginal microbiota remained constant. A subanalysis of women with Lactobacillus spp dominance before antibiotic exposure showed that erythromycin treatment associated with a shift toward intermediate or dysbiotic community structure. In contrast, in samples collected

---

Fig. 1. Individual patient-level analysis of paired vaginal microbiota samples before and after PPROM, before erythromycin treatment. (A) Stacked bar chart displaying percentage abundance of the top 25 bacterial genera demonstrating transition from a Lactobacillus spp–dominant community to a Lactobacillus spp deplete community in 3/8 (37.5%), persistence of a Lactobacillus spp deplete community in 4/12 (25%), and maintenance of a Lactobacillus spp–dominant community in 5/12 (41%) of individuals. (B) Richness of microbial communities increases significantly following PPROM (P = .048). Further details on patient samples and methodology are presented elsewhere.[62]

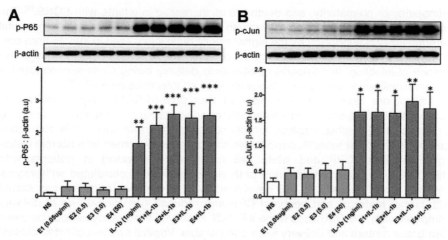

Fig. 2. Erythromycin does not inhibit inflammatory pathway activation in amniocytes. Western blot analysis of the phosphorylated (activated) forms of the subunits of inflammatory transcription factors (*A*) NFκB (P65) and (*B*) AP-1 (cJun) in amniocytes cell cultures at 1 hour, following no treatment (NS), treatment with erythromycin alone at 0.05 (E1), 0.5 (E2), 5.0 (E3), and 50 μg/mL (E4), IL-1β(1 ng/mL) alone, and IL-1β (1 ng/mL) after 2 hours pretreatment with 0.05, 0.5, 5.0, and 50 μg/mL erythromycin, n = 5. Experimental details are provided elsewhere.[85] *P<0.05, **P<0.01, ***P<0.001.

from women with *Lactobacillus* spp depletion, erythromycin treatment was associated with a reduction in both richness and diversity despite unchanged bacterial load. Similar results were observed in paired samples taken before and 48 hours after erythromycin treatment. These results further indicate that oral dosing of erythromycin leads to a vaginal lumen concentration sufficient to impede colonization of *Lactobacillus* spp but not to substantially impact growth of potential pathogenic species.

Even if not the primary driver of dysbiosis, these data show that erythromycin fails to improve the composition of the vaginal microbiome by eradicating potential pathogens or reducing overall bacterial load and appears to be especially detrimental for individuals with a *Lactobacillus* spp–dominated microbiome. Further evidence supporting this conclusion has since been reported in an Australian retrospective cohort study of mother-infant dyads who delivered at less than 30 weeks of gestation following PPROM.[87] The investigators reported that women receiving erythromycin had increased incidence of antimicrobial-resistant Gram-negative organisms on placental swabs and that this treatment strategy may promote selection of antimicrobial-resistant Gram-negative organisms and increase risk of Gram-negative early-onset sepsis.

VAGINAL MICROBIOTA AND NEONATAL OUTCOME FOLLOWING PRETERM PREMATURE RUPTURE OF MEMBRANES

Clinical and histologic chorioamnionitis and funisitis are the major risk factors for early-onset neonatal sepsis (EONS) in the preterm infant. Many studies have associated perinatal infection and inflammation, chorioamnionitis, and EONS with brain injury, including periventricular leukomalacia (PVL), neurodevelopmental delay, and cerebral palsy. EONS and exposure to intrauterine inflammation from chorioamnionitis are also associated with an increased risk of development of bronchopulmonary dysplasia (BPD) in preterm infants. Incidences of BPD, PVL, intraventricular hemorrhage, retinopathy of prematurity, and death are all increased in infants with EONS.[88] The concept that infection/inflammation-driven PTB also contributes to fetal or neonatal cerebral injury is supported by the higher risk of brain injury seen in infants born preterm with PPROM or spontaneous onset of labor, which is associated with high frequency of infection. In comparison, iatrogenic delivery owing to severe intrauterine growth restriction is very rarely associated with an infectious cause.[89,90]

The authors have previously reported that post-PPROM, vaginal microbiota composition before delivery in women with chorioamnionitis with funisitis is enriched for *Prevotella*, *Sneathia*, *Peptostreptococcus*, and *Catonella* spp and is characterized by reduced *Lactobacillus* spp levels compared with women with normal histology.[62] Maternal CRP and white cell count were elevated in patients with chorioamnionitis with funisitis, and both were significantly correlated with vaginal bacterial alpha diversity. EONS developed in 22% of cases and was associated with higher maternal and neonatal CRP and reduced gestational age at delivery compared with PPROM cases without EONS. However, the latency periods between membrane rupture and delivery were comparable. Vaginal swabs collected closest to the time of delivery were enriched for *Catonella* spp and *Sneathia* spp in cases developing EONS, whereas *L crispatus* was overrepresented in the maternal vaginal microbiota of neonates who did not develop EONS. Other species previously associated with EONS, including *Streptococcus agalactiae*, *Fusobacterium nucleatum*, and *Escherichia coli*, were frequently observed in vaginal samples collected from EONS-complicated pregnancies but not in samples isolated from uncomplicated controls. The data remained similar when analysis was undertaken only for those mothers who delivered at 28 weeks or sooner to account for the differences in gestational age at delivery.

CERVICAL CERCLAGE, LARGE LOOP EXCISION OF THE TRANSFORMATION ZONE OF THE CERVIX, CERVICAL INTRAEPITHELIAL NEOPLASIA, AND PRETERM PREMATURE RUPTURE OF MEMBRANES

A prepregnancy history of large loop excision of the transformation zone of the cervix (LLETZ), or cone biopsy to treat cervical intraepithelial neoplasia (CIN), or of trachelectomy for early cervical cancer is a significant risk factor for PPROM. There is a small background increase in the rate of PTB in women with untreated CIN, but the principal risk of PTB relates to the degree of tissue destruction with a "depth-dependent" relationship between depth of excision of cervical tissue and subsequent PTB risk.[91] A recent Cochrane review reported that the overall risk of PTB in women with a prior LLETZ of any size of depth is 9.5%, whereas the risk of PPROM is 8%.[92] This finding converts to relative risk of 1.8 for PTB and 2.4 for PPROM compared with background rates. The authors' own experience of managing a large number of pregnancies complicated by cold knife cone biopsy, LLETZ, or trachelectomy is that in the background population about 40% of women who deliver preterm do so following PPROM, but this increases to around 80% in women with a prior LLETZ and almost 100% in women with a prior trachelectomy (Bennett PR, unpublished data, 2020).

CIN is associated with an increased prevalence of vaginal microbiota characterized by high diversity and low levels of *Lactobacillus* spp, and the authors have previously shown that increasing severity of CIN associates with decreasing relative abundance of *Lactobacillus* spp.[93] A subsequent study of adolescent and young women with histologically confirmed, untreated CIN2 lesions showed that women with *Lactobacillus* dominance of vaginal microbiota at baseline are more likely to have regressive disease at 12 months.[94] It is therefore plausible that women with

CIN or a previous LLETZ may be at increased risk of PPROM during a subsequent pregnancy because of an increased rate of vaginal dysbiosis. There are currently no published studies of either the effect of LLETZ on the vaginal microbiota or the effect of pregnancy upon the vaginal microbiota in women who have had LLETZ.

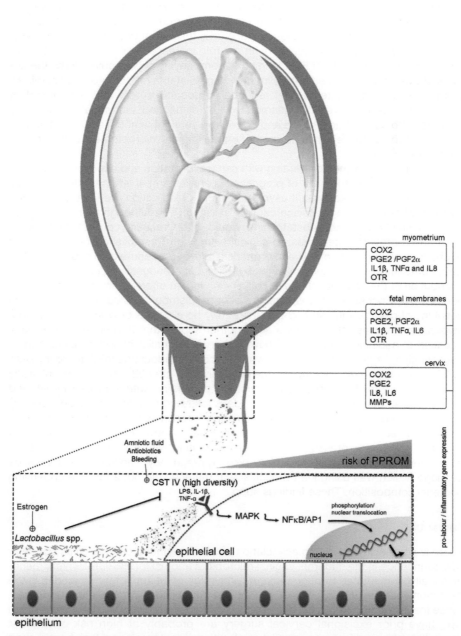

Fig. 3. The role vaginal microbiota play in mediating inflammatory pathway activation leading to PPROM. IL-1β, interleukin-1β; LPS, lipopolysaccharide; MAPK, mitogen-activated protein kinase; TNF-α, tumor necrosis factor.

The authors have, however, seen excellent outcomes in women with a prior LLETZ who are managed by surveillance of cervical length during pregnancy with targeted cervical cerclage.[95] It can be calculated that the PTB rate in women managed using this strategy is 8.4%, compared with an overall national PTB rate of 7.8%. However, these good outcomes are dependent on the type of suture material used to perform cerclage. The PTB rate was 15% in those women whose cerclage was performed using monofilament material but 40% in those in whom a braided suture (Mersilene) was used. In an earlier large case-control study, the use of braided suture material for cerclage was found to associate with a 3-fold increase in intrauterine fetal death and a doubling in the rate of PTB.[57] In an accompanying prospective study, the authors showed that a braided suture induces a persistent shift toward vaginal microbiome dysbiosis characterized by reduced *Lactobacillus* spp and enrichment of pathobionts, associated with inflammatory cytokine and interstitial collagenase excretion into cervicovaginal fluid and premature cervical remodeling. Monofilament suture had comparatively minimal impact on the vaginal microbiome and its interactions with the host.

Management of women presenting with cervical dilatation and exposed fetal membranes in the second trimester of pregnancy is challenging. If left untreated most will deliver within 2-3 weeks, even if asymptomatic at presentation, frequently preceded by PPROM and resulting in miscarriage or extreme PTB. Although management remains contentious, many obstetricians would offer 'rescue' cervical cerclage in such cases provided there was no clinical evidence of established preterm labour or chorioamnionitis. One of the significant risks of this procedure is to cause PPROM. Data from a large cohort study reported by Pereira et al suggested a possible bimodal distribution of the gestational age of delivery in women offered cerclage in this situation.[96] Ehsanipoor et al., propose that this bimodal distribution is due to the underlying aetiology of cervical dilation and that there may be a subset of women with a more favourable outcome after cerclage and another subset that is likely to deliver early because of subclinical infection.[97] have observed a similar bimodal distribution of the gestational age of delivery in our own practice, with about one third delivering prior to 24 completed weeks, and about one half delivering after 32 weeks. A recent study of vaginal microbiota composition in women presenting with a dilated cervix and exposed fetal membranes before and 10 days following rescue cervical cerclage reported reduced *Lactobacillus* spp. relative abundance in 40% of cases prior to cerclage compared to 10% of gestational age-matched controls.cerclage[74]. *Gardnerella vaginalis* was over-represented in women presenting with symptoms and those in whom rescue cerclage failed to usefully prolong pregnancy. The insertion of a rescue cerclage, which was using inert monofilament material, did not affect the underlying bacterial composition. These findings supp

SUMMARY

There is good evidence for an association between reduced *Lactobacillus* spp relative abundance in the maternal vaginal microbiota and risk of PPROM, which, mechanistically, is mediated through untimely activation of inflammatory cascades in the gestational tissues (**Fig. 3**). Cases of PPROM appear to be divisible into 2 groups: those that are linked to vaginal dysbiosis, and those that have other causes. Women who have prior excisional cervical surgery are probably at high risk of PPROM through mechanical factors and will do well with cervical cerclage if they have a short cervix, although choice of suture material may affect outcomes. In most cases of PPROM linked to vaginal dysbiosis, reduced *Lactobacillus* spp relative abundance develops close to the time of membrane rupture, although dysbiosis at any gestational age increases the risk. The event of PPROM itself may change the vaginal microbiota in some women through direct effects of amniotic fluid; however, antibiotic therapy appears to have a greater effect. In women with *Lactobacillus* spp deletion at the time of PPROM, antibiotics may have a beneficial effect on bacterial load, but antibiotics appear to damage optimal vaginal microbiota communities by selectively targeting *Lactobacillus* spp Both chorioamnionitis and early-onset neonatal sepsis, which are risk factors for developmental delay, cerebral palsy, and a range of other adverse neonatal outcomes, are increased where the vaginal microbiota are *Lactobacillus* spp depleted close to the time of delivery. It is now time to reconsider the role of antibiotic therapy in PPROM, and to develop strategies to allow targeted rather than universal therapy. Many studies have identified a role for *L crispatus* as protective against PTB, which opens the way for preventative strategies involving live therapeutics.

CLINICS CARE POINTS

- A *Lactobacillus* spp depleted microbiome at any gestational age is a risk factor for PPROM, however current antibiotic therapies do not appear to change this risk. Many studies have identified a protective role for *L crispatus* against PTB, which opens the way for preventative strategies involving live therapeutics.
- Cases of PPROM may be divisible into at least two broad phenotypes, some infection-mediated and associated with an adverse vaginal microbiota, and other non-infectious aetiologies. The former associates with increased risk of chorioamnionitis and adverse neonatal outcomes.
- Women with a previous LLETZ have an increased risk of preterm birth which can be largely mitigated by cervical cerclage targeted at those with a short cervix.
- The suture material used for cervical cerclage may adversely affect the vaginal microbiota. Insertion of a monofilament suture material appears to be a better choice than a braided material.

ACKNOWLEDGMENTS

This work was supported by the March of Dimes European Prematurity Research Centre, NIHR BRC at Imperial Healthcare NHS Trust, the Medical Research Council and Genesis Research Trust.

DISCLOSURE

P.R. Bennett and D.A. MacIntyre are named inventors on patents held by Imperial College relating to biomarker discovery in preterm birth. P.R. Bennett has been a paid or unpaid consultant to Samsung, GSK, ObsEva in relation to commercial preterm birth research.

REFERENCES

1. Causes of child mortality. Available at: http://www.who.int/gho/child_health/mortality/causes/en/. Accessed July 7, 2016.
2. Parry S, Strauss JF 3rd. Premature rupture of the fetal membranes. N Engl J Med 1998;338(10):663–70.
3. Liu L, Oza S, Hogan D, et al. Global, regional, and national causes of child mortality in 2000-13, with projections to inform post-2015 priorities: an updated systematic analysis. Lancet 2015;385(9966):430–40.

4. Lamont RF, Duncan SLB, Mandal D, et al. Intravaginal clindamycin to reduce pre-term birth in women with abnormal genital tract flora. Obstet Gynecol 2003; 101(3):516–22.

5. Pappas A, Kendrick DE, Shankaran S, et al. Chorioamnionitis and early childhood outcomes among extremely low-gestational-age neonates. JAMA Pediatr 2014; 168(2):137–47.

6. De Martino SJ, Mahoudeau I, Brettes JP, et al. Peripartum bacteremias due to Leptotrichia amnionii and Sneathia sanguinegens, rare causes of fever during and after delivery. J Clin Microbiol 2004;42(12):5940–3.

7. Karat C, Madhivanan P, Krupp K, et al. The clinical and microbiological correlates of premature rupture of membranes. Indian J Med Microbiol 2006;24(4):283–5.

8. Furman B, Shoham-Vardi I, Bashiri A, et al. Clinical significance and outcome of preterm prelabor rupture of membranes: population-based study. Eur J Obstet Gynecol Reprod Biol 2000;92(2):209–16.

9. Flynn CA, Helwig AL, Meurer LN. Bacterial vaginosis in pregnancy and the risk of prematurity: a meta-analysis. J Fam Pract 1999;48(11):885–92.

10. McGregor JA, French JI, Seo K. Premature rupture of membranes and bacterial vaginosis. Am J Obstet Gynecol 1993;169(2 Pt 2):463–6.

11. Donders GG, Van Calsteren K, Bellen G, et al. Predictive value for preterm birth of abnormal vaginal flora, bacterial vaginosis and aerobic vaginitis during the first trimester of pregnancy. BJOG 2009;116(10):1315–24.

12. Coleman JS, Gaydos CA, Witter F. Trichomonas vaginalis vaginitis in obstetrics and gynecology practice: new concepts and controversies. Obstet Gynecol Surv 2013;68(1):43–50.

13. Chandiramani M, Bennett PR, Brown R, et al. Vaginal microbiome–pregnant host interactions determine a significant proportion of preterm labour. Fetal Matern Med Rev 2014;25(01):73–8.

14. Kanayama N, Terao T, Horiuchi K. The role of human neutrophil elastase in the premature rupture of membranes. Asia Oceania J Obstet Gynaecol 1988;14(3): 389–97.

15. Fortunato SJ, Menon R, Lombardi SJ. Role of tumor necrosis factor-alpha in the premature rupture of membranes and preterm labor pathways. Am J Obstet Gynecol 2002;187(5):1159–62.

16. Shobokshi A, Shaarawy M. Maternal serum and amniotic fluid cytokines in patients with preterm premature rupture of membranes with and without intrauterine infection. Int J Gynaecol Obstet 2002;79(3):209–15.

17. Helmig BR, Romero R, Espinoza J, et al. Neutrophil elastase and secretory leukocyte protease inhibitor in prelabor rupture of membranes, parturition and intra-amniotic infection. J Matern Fetal Neonatal Med 2002;12(4):237–46.

18. Romero R, Dey SK, Fisher SJ. Preterm labor: one syndrome, many causes. Science 2014;345:760–5.

19. Fortner KB, Grotegut CA, Ransom CE, et al. Bacteria localization and chorion thinning among preterm premature rupture of membranes. PLoS One 2014; 9(1):e83338.

20. Rocha G, Proenca E, Quintas C, et al. Chorioamnionitis and brain damage in the preterm newborn. J Matern Fetal Neonatal Med 2007;20(10):745–9.

21. Lu H, Wang Q, Lu J, et al. Risk factors for intraventricular hemorrhage in preterm infants born at 34 weeks of gestation or less following preterm premature rupture of membranes. J Stroke Cerebrovasc Dis 2016;25(4):807–12.

22. Vigneswaran R. Infection and preterm birth: evidence of a common causal relationship with bronchopulmonary dysplasia and cerebral palsy. Paediatr Child Health 2000;36(4):293–6.
23. Yoon BH, Romero R, Park JS, et al. Fetal exposure to an intra-amniotic inflammation and the development of cerebral palsy at the age of three years. Am J Obstet Gynecol 2000;182(3):675–81.
24. Drassinower D, Friedman AM, Obican SG, et al. Prolonged latency of preterm premature rupture of membranes and risk of cerebral palsy. J Matern Fetal Neonatal Med 2015;29(17):2748–52.
25. van Dillen J, Zwart J, Schutte J, et al. Maternal sepsis: epidemiology, etiology and outcome. Curr Opin Infect Dis 2010;23(3):249–54.
26. Puri K, Taft DH, Ambalavanan N, et al. Association of chorioamnionitis with aberrant neonatal gut colonization and adverse clinical outcomes. PLoS One 2016; 11(9):e0162734.
27. Brocklehurst P, Gordon A, Heatley E, et al. Antibiotics for treating bacterial vaginosis in pregnancy. Cochrane Database Syst Rev 2013;(1):Cd000262.
28. Menon R, Yu J, Basanta-Henry P, et al. Short fetal leukocyte telomere length and preterm prelabor rupture of the membranes. PloS one 2012;7(2):e31136.
29. Mohan AR, Sooranna SR, Lindstrom TM, et al. The effect of mechanical stretch on cyclooxygenase type 2 expression and activator protein-1 and nuclear factor-kappaB activity in human amnion cells. Endocrinology 2007;148(4):1850–7.
30. Cummings LA, Kurosawa K, Hoogestraat DR, et al. Clinical next generation sequencing outperforms standard microbiological culture for characterizing polymicrobial samples. Clin Chem 2016;62(11):1465–73.
31. Marchesi JR, Ravel J. The vocabulary of microbiome research: a proposal. Microbiome 2015;3:31.
32. Shreiner AB, Kao JY, Young VB. The gut microbiome in health and in disease. Curr Opin Gastroenterol 2015;31(1):69–75.
33. MacIntyre DA, Sykes L, Bennett PB. The human female urogenital microbiome: complexity in normality. Emerg Top Life Sci 2017;1(4):363–72.
34. de Goffau MC, Lager S, Sovio U, et al. Human placenta has no microbiome but can contain potential pathogens. Nature 2019;572(7769):329–34.
35. Aagaard K, Ma J, Antony KM, et al. The placenta harbors a unique microbiome. Sci Transl Med 2014;6(237):237ra265.
36. Chakravorty S, Helb D, Burday M, et al. A detailed analysis of 16S ribosomal RNA gene segments for the diagnosis of pathogenic bacteria. J Microbiol Methods 2007;69(2):330–9.
37. Dominguez-Bello MG, Costello EK, Contreras M, et al. Delivery mode shapes the acquisition and structure of the initial microbiota across multiple body habitats in newborns. Proc Natl Acad Sci U S A 2010;107(26):11971–5.
38. Hill GB, St Claire KK, Gutman LT. Anaerobes predominate among the vaginal microflora of prepubertal girls. Clin Infect Dis 1995;20(Suppl 2):S269–70.
39. Linhares IM, Summers PR, Larsen B, et al. Contemporary perspectives on vaginal pH and lactobacilli. Am J Obstet Gynecol 2011;204:120.e1-5.
40. Hickey RJ, Zhou X, Pierson JD, et al. Understanding vaginal microbiome complexity from an ecological perspective. Transl Res 2012;160(4):267–82.
41. Zheng J, Ganzle MG, Lin XB, et al. Diversity and dynamics of bacteriocins from human microbiome. Environ Microbiol 2015;17(6):2133–43.
42. Velraeds MM, van de Belt-Gritter B, van der Mei HC, et al. Interference in initial adhesion of uropathogenic bacteria and yeasts to silicone rubber by a Lactobacillus acidophilus biosurfactant. J Med Microbiol 1998;47(12):1081–5.

43. Antonio MA, Rabe LK, Hillier SL. Colonization of the rectum by Lactobacillus species and decreased risk of bacterial vaginosis. J Infect Dis 2005;192(3):394–8.

44. Eschenbach DA, Davick PR, Williams BL, et al. Prevalence of hydrogen peroxide-producing Lactobacillus species in normal women and women with bacterial vaginosis. J Clin Microbiol 1989;27(2):251–6.

45. Ness RB, Hillier SL, Kip KE, et al. Bacterial vaginosis and risk of pelvic inflammatory disease. Obstet Gynecol 2004;104(4):761–9.

46. Wang S, Wang Q, Yang E, et al. Antimicrobial compounds produced by vaginal lactobacillus crispatus are able to strongly inhibit candida albicans growth, hyphal formation and regulate virulence-related gene expressions. Front Microbiol 2017;8:564.

47. Borgdorff H, Tsivtsivadze E, Verhelst R, et al. Lactobacillus-dominated cervicovaginal microbiota associated with reduced HIV/STI prevalence and genital HIV viral load in African women. ISME J 2014;8(9):1781–93.

48. Ravel J, Gajer P, Abdo Z, et al. Vaginal microbiome of reproductive-age women. Proc Natl Acad Sci U S A 2011;108(Suppl 1):4680–7.

49. Fettweis JM, Brooks JP, Serrano MG, et al. Differences in vaginal microbiome in African American women versus women of European ancestry. Microbiology 2014;160(Pt 10):2272–82.

50. MacIntyre DA, Chandiramani M, Lee YS, et al. The vaginal microbiome during pregnancy and the postpartum period in a European population. Sci Rep 2015;5:8988.

51. Romero R, Hassan SS, Gajer P, et al. The composition and stability of the vaginal microbiota of normal pregnant women is different from that of non-pregnant women. Microbiome 2014;2(1):4.

52. Roy EJ, Mackay R. The concentration of oestrogens in blood during pregnancy. J Obstet Gynaecol Br Emp 1962;69:13–7.

53. Aagaard K, Riehle K, Ma J, et al. A metagenomic approach to characterization of the vaginal microbiome signature in pregnancy. PLoS One 2012;7(6):e36466.

54. DiGiulio DB, Callahan BJ, McMurdie PJ, et al. Temporal and spatial variation of the human microbiota during pregnancy. Proc Natl Acad Sci U S A 2015; 112(35):11060–5.

55. Peelen MJ, Luef BM, Lamont RF, et al. The influence of the vaginal microbiota on preterm birth: a systematic review and recommendations for a minimum dataset for future research. Placenta 2019;79:30–9.

56. Hyman RW, Fukushima M, Jiang H, et al. Diversity of the vaginal microbiome correlates with preterm birth. Reprod Sci 2014;21(1):32–40.

57. Kindinger LM, MacIntyre DA, Lee YS, et al. Relationship between vaginal microbial dysbiosis, inflammation, and pregnancy outcomes in cervical cerclage. Sci Transl Med 2016;8(350):350ra102.

58. Romero R, Hassan SS, Gajer P, et al. The vaginal microbiota of pregnant women who subsequently have spontaneous preterm labor and delivery and those with a normal delivery at term. Microbiome 2014;2:18.

59. Stout MJ, Zhou Y, Wylie KM, et al. Early pregnancy vaginal microbiome trends and preterm birth. Am J Obstet Gynecol 2017;217(3):356.e1-18.

60. MacIntyre DA, Bennett PR. Microbial signatures of preterm birth. In: Koren O, Rautava S, editors. The human microbiome in early life. Elsevier; 2020. Available at. https://www.elsevier.com/books/the-human-microbiome-in-early-life/koren/ 978-0-12-818097-6.

61. Brown RG, Al-Memar M, Marchesi JR, et al. Establishment of vaginal microbiota composition in early pregnancy and its association with subsequent preterm prelabor rupture of the fetal membranes. Transl Res 2019;207:30–43.
62. Brown RG, Marchesi JR, Lee YS, et al. Vaginal dysbiosis increases risk of preterm fetal membrane rupture, neonatal sepsis and is exacerbated by erythromycin. BMC Med 2018;16(1):9.
63. Callahan BJ, DiGiulio DB, Goltsman DSA, et al. Replication and refinement of a vaginal microbial signature of preterm birth in two racially distinct cohorts of US women. Proc Natl Acad Sci U S A 2017;114(37):9966–71.
64. Elovitz MA, Gajer P, Riis V, et al. Cervicovaginal microbiota and local immune response modulate the risk of spontaneous preterm delivery. Nat Commun 2019;10(1):1305.
65. Fettweis JM, Serrano MG, Brooks JP, et al. The vaginal microbiome and preterm birth. Nat Med 2019;25(6):1012–21.
66. Freitas AC, Bocking A, Hill JE, et al. Increased richness and diversity of the vaginal microbiota and spontaneous preterm birth. Microbiome 2018;6(1):117.
67. Kindinger LM, Bennett PR, Lee YS, et al. The interaction between vaginal microbiota, cervical length, and vaginal progesterone treatment for preterm birth risk. Microbiome 2017;5(1):6.
68. Tabatabaei N, Eren AM, Barreiro LB, et al. Vaginal microbiome in early pregnancy and subsequent risk of spontaneous preterm birth: a case-control study. BJOG 2019;126(3):349–58.
69. Stafford GP, Parker JL, Amabebe E, et al. Spontaneous preterm birth is associated with differential expression of vaginal metabolites by lactobacilli-dominated microflora. Front Physiol 2017;8:615.
70. Hocevar K, Maver A, Vidmar Simic M, et al. Vaginal microbiome signature is associated with spontaneous preterm delivery. Front Med (Lausanne) 2019;6:201.
71. Nelson DB, Shin H, Wu J, et al. The gestational vaginal microbiome and spontaneous preterm birth among nulliparous African American women. Am J Perinatol 2016;33(9):887–93.
72. Brown RG, Chan D, Terzidou V, et al. Prospective observational study of vaginal microbiota pre- and post-rescue cervical cerclage. BJOG 2019;126(7):916–25.
73. Al-Memar M, Bobdiwala S, Fourie H, et al. The association between vaginal bacterial composition and miscarriage: a nested case-control study. BJOG 2020; 127(2):264–74.
74. Al-Memar M, Vaulet T, Fourie H, et al. Early-pregnancy events and subsequent antenatal, delivery and neonatal outcomes: prospective cohort study. Ultrasound Obstet Gynecol 2019;54(4):530–7.
75. Kacerovsky M, Vrbacky F, Kutova R, et al. Cervical microbiota in women with preterm prelabor rupture of membranes. PLoS One 2015;10(5):e0126884.
76. Paramel Jayaprakash T, Wagner EC, van Schalkwyk J, et al. High diversity and variability in the vaginal microbiome in women following preterm premature rupture of membranes (PPROM): a prospective cohort study. PLoS One 2016; 11(11):e0166794.
77. Varrey A, Romero R, Panaitescu B, et al. Human beta-defensin-1: a natural antimicrobial peptide present in amniotic fluid that is increased in spontaneous preterm labor with intra-amniotic infection. Am J Reprod Immunol 2018;80(4): e13031.
78. Ramsey PS, Nuthalapaty FS, Lu G, et al. Contemporary management of preterm premature rupture of membranes (PPROM): a survey of maternal-fetal medicine providers. Am J Obstet Gynecol 2004;191(4):1497–502.

79. Kenyon SL, Taylor DJ, Tarnow-Mordi W, et al. Broad-spectrum antibiotics for pre-term, prelabour rupture of fetal membranes: the ORACLE I randomised trial. ORACLE Collaborative Group. Lancet 2001;357(9261):979–88.

80. Iliopoulou A, Thin RN, Turner P. Fluorimetric and microbiological assays of eryth-romycin concentrations in plasma and vaginal washings. Br J Vener Dis 1981; 57(4):263–7.

81. Kuriyama T, Williams DW, Yanagisawa M, et al. Antimicrobial susceptibility of 800 anaerobic isolates from patients with dentoalveolar infection to 13 oral antibiotics. Oral Microbiol Immunol 2007;22(4):285–8.

82. Harwich MD Jr, Serrano MG, Fettweis JM, et al. Genomic sequence analysis and characterization of Sneathia amnii sp. nov. BMC Genomics 2012;13(Suppl 8):S4.

83. Koyama H, Geddes DM. Erythromycin and diffuse panbronchiolitis. Thorax 1997; 52(10):915–8.

84. Desaki M, Okazaki H, Sunazuka T, et al. Molecular mechanisms of anti-inflammatory action of erythromycin in human bronchial epithelial cells: possible role in the signaling pathway that regulates nuclear factor-kappaB activation. Antimicrob Agents Chemother 2004;48(5):1581–5.

85. Brown RG. The vaginal microbiome in preterm prelabour rupture of the fetal membranes. London: Department of Surgery and Cancer, Imperial College London; 2018.

86. Baldwin EA, Walther-Antonio M, MacLean AM, et al. Persistent microbial dysbio-sis in preterm premature rupture of membranes from onset until delivery. PeerJ 2015;3:e1398.

87. Axford SB, Andersen CC, Stark MJ. Patterns of placental antimicrobial resistance in preterm birth before 30 completed weeks gestation complicated by preterm prelabour rupture of membranes. Aust N Z J Obstet Gynaecol 2020;60(4): 509–13.

88. Simonsen KA, Anderson-Berry AL, Delair SF, et al. Early-onset neonatal sepsis. Clin Microbiol Rev 2014;27(1):21–47.

89. Dammann O, Allred EN, Veelken N. Increased risk of spastic diplegia among very low birth weight children after preterm labor or prelabor rupture of membranes. J Pediatr 1998;132(3 Pt 1):531–5.

90. Verma U, Tejani N, Klein S, et al. Obstetric antecedents of intraventricular hemor-rhage and periventricular leukomalacia in the low-birth-weight neonate. Am J Ob-stet Gynecol 1997;176(2):275–81.

91. Kyrgiou M, Athanasiou A, Paraskevaidi M, et al. Adverse obstetric outcomes after local treatment for cervical preinvasive and early invasive disease according to cone depth: systematic review and meta-analysis. BMJ 2016;354:i3633.

92. Kyrgiou M, Athanasiou A, Kalliala IEJ, et al. Obstetric outcomes after conserva-tive treatment for cervical intraepithelial lesions and early invasive disease. Co-chrane Database Syst Rev 2017;(11):CD012847.

93. Mitra A, MacIntyre DA, Lee YS, et al. Cervical intraepithelial neoplasia disease progression is associated with increased vaginal microbiome diversity. Sci Rep 2015;5:16865.

94. Mitra A, MacIntyre DA, Ntritsos G, et al. The vaginal microbiota associates with the regression of untreated cervical intraepithelial neoplasia 2 lesions. Nat Com-mun 2020;11(1):1999.

95. Kindinger LM, Kyrgiou M, MacIntyre DA, et al. Preterm birth prevention post-conization: a model of cervical length screening with targeted cerclage. PLoS One 2016;11(11):e0163793.

96. Pereira L, Cotter A, Gomez R, et al. Expectant management compared with physical examination-indicated cerclage (EM-PEC) in selected women with a dilated cervix at 14(0/7)-25(6/7) weeks: results from the EM-PEC international cohort study. Am J Obstet Gynecol 2007;197(5):483.e1-8.

97. Ehsanipoor RM, Seligman NS, Saccone G, et al. Physical examination-indicated cerclage: a systematic review and meta-analysis. Obstet Gynecol 2015;126(1): 125–35.

Mechanism of Human Fetal Membrane Biomechanical Weakening, Rupture and Potential Targets for Therapeutic Intervention

Check for updates

Deepak Kumar, MD[a],*, Robert M. Moore, MS[a],
Brian M. Mercer, MD[b], Joseph M. Mansour, PhD[c],
John J. Moore, MD[a,b]

KEYWORDS

- Fetal membranes • Biomechanical weakening • pPROM • TNF • Thrombin
- GM-CSF • Progesterone • α-Lipoic acid

KEY POINTS

- Toward the end of gestation, the human fetal membranes (FM) develop a biochemically mediated physiologic weak zone overlying the cervix due to extracellular matrix remodeling and cellular apoptosis.
- In our novel in vitro model of FM weakening, tumor necrosis factor (TNF) (modeling infection-inflammation) and thrombin (modeling decidual bleeding-abruption), major determinants of preterm premature rupture of the membranes, induce FM weakening and biochemical changes in human FM explants, mimicking the physiologic weak zone.
- Granulocyte-macrophage colony-stimulating factor (GM-CSF) is a critical common intermediate in TNF and thrombin-induced FM weakening. GM-CSF is both necessary and sufficient for the FM weakening process.

Continued

Funding: NIH HD48476, March of Dimes 21-FY11-9 and Burroughs Wellcome Fund 1015024 to J. J. Moore.
[a] Department of Pediatrics, MetroHealth Medical Center, Case Western Reserve University, 2500 MetroHealth Drive, Cleveland, OH 44109, USA; [b] Department of Reproductive Biology, MetroHealth Medical Center, Case Western Reserve University, 2500 MetroHealth Drive, Cleveland, OH 44109, USA; [c] Mechanical and Aerospace Engineering, Case Western Reserve University, Glennan 617, Cleveland, OH 44106, USA
* Corresponding author. Case Western Reserve School of Medicine, MetroHealth Campus, 2500 MetroHealth Drive, Cleveland, OH 44109.
E-mail address: dkumar@metrohealth.org

Obstet Gynecol Clin N Am 47 (2020) 523–544
https://doi.org/10.1016/j.ogc.2020.08.010
0889-8545/20/© 2020 Elsevier Inc. All rights reserved.

Continued

- TNF, thrombin, and GM-CSF primarily act on choriodecidua, and not the major FM strength determinant amnion, to cause FM weakening. GM-CSF acts on decidual monocytes-macrophages to induce proteases and inhibit protease inhibitors.
- Progestogens (progesterone, medroxyprogesterone acetate and 17α-hydroxyprogesterone) inhibit both GM-CSF production and its downstream action, but 17α-hydroxy-progesterone caproate only inhibits GM-CSF production (not GM-CSF action), which may explain its relative lack of efficacy in clinical use.

BACKGROUND

Preterm birth is the major (60%–70%) cause of infant mortality and morbidity in the United States.[1,2] Preterm premature rupture of the membranes (pPROM) causes as much as 50% of potentially preventable preterm births.[3,4] One pathway to significantly decrease the infant mortality rate in the United States is to decrease preterm birth. Infection, inflammation, and decidual bleeding are major drivers of pPROM.[5] Therapies to prevent preterm birth are confounded by substantial gaps in understanding of the mechanisms of fetal membrane (FM) weakening and rupture.[6]

A limitation to understanding pPROM is the lack of animal models. Nearly all studies of FM biology and physiology pursue a cell biology or tissue histology–based approach, which can only provide limited insight into the structural mechanisms of FM tissue weakening, which leads to pPROM. Therefore, any presumed etiology of FM rupture must ultimately be tested with a model in which actual changes to FM physical properties can be demonstrated. We have integrated biochemical and histologic studies with biomechanical testing of FM strength to develop a model system to study human FM weakening process.[7,8] In this review, we first discuss key concepts into the mechanism of human FM biomechanical weakening and rupture. Second, we discuss how models have been used to screen potential targets for therapeutic intervention to prevent pPROM.[6–8]

FETAL MEMBRANE RUPTURE AND THE ONSET OF LABOR

Most labor at term begins with uterine contractions followed by spontaneous rupture of the FM (SROM), or by artificial rupture (AROM). In 10% of term births and approximately 40% of preterm births SROM precedes labor contractions.[9] Acute inflammation, infection, and decidual hemorrhage are highly associated with pPROM and preterm birth. This correlates with the presence of inflammatory changes seen histologically in 26% to 50% of placentas following pPROM.[10,11]

The FM undergo cyclical stretch during in response to uterine contractions that have a complex effect on FM strength. Repetitive stretch is considered important in membrane weakening because the FM is noted to rupture with labor contractions that vary in intensity.[12] Conversely, FM subjected to cyclical stretching to simulate labor contractions did not weaken but paradoxically caused the membranes to rupture at a significantly higher force.[13] Stretch forces alone do not appear to be adequate to rupture FM without some form of preweakening.[14]

Normally, in preparation for parturition, the FM region overlying the cervix weakens and develops morphologic changes, such as collagen remodeling and cellular apoptosis.[15–23] This developmental peri-cervical focal FM area is a physiologic weak zone where spontaneous FM rupture typically occurs.[15,16]

Proinflammatory cytokines normally increase in amniotic fluid with gestation and increase acutely with rupture of membranes. They are induced in infection and abruption causing FM apoptosis along with induction and activation of matrix metalloproteinases (MMPs).[19,24–32] Synergy between MMP activation and apoptotic changes leads to FM weakening and rupture.[24,32,33] Presumably MMP activation leading to collagen degradation and proteoglycan disruption leads to weakening of FM by decreasing tensile strength or by precluding the ability of the tissue to repair damage.

MEASUREMENT OF FETAL MEMBRANE STRENGTH

Human FMs are a complex tissue and thus determination of their biomechanical "strength" is not straightforward. Three main testing methodologies have been used with FM[8]: (1) tensile testing (membrane strip clamped at 2 ends is pulled apart); (2) burst testing (air or fluid pressure applied to membrane clamped in a ring); and (3) puncture testing (a spherical metal probe used to displace the central portion of a membrane fragment clamped in a ring). Using any of these methods, a force (applied to the tissue) versus displacement (movement of the tissue in response to the force) curve is generated to describe the biomechanical properties of the FM. Rupture Strength (force required to rupture), Stiffness (related to elasticity), and Work to Rupture (Energy required to rupture), especially Rupture Strength, are the main parameters of interest[8] (**Fig. 1**). Our testing apparatus (described in more detail as follows) uses the puncture mode because puncture causes a more physiologic 2-dimensional stretching of the FM (unlike Tensile testing, which is 1 dimensional) and it allows small fragments of the FM to be rapidly tested (unlike burst testing).[7,8]

Most studies of the FM report that the amnion is stronger than the chorion. In addition, FMs have viscoelastic properties and tissue strength is nonhomogeneous over its surface. There are contradictory reports of whether the amnion or the chorion ruptures first.[13,34,35] FM biomechanical strength characteristics are influenced by many biochemical factors including MMPs (2, 3, 9, 10), tissue inhibitors of

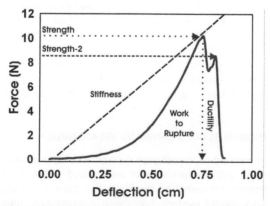

Fig. 1. Idealized FM force-deflection curve. Force in Newtons, Deflection in centimeters. Parameters include the following: rupture strength is the peak of the curve (Strength); rupture of the amnion is (Strength-2); Work to rupture is the area under the curve; Stiffness is the slope of the line labeled Stiffness; Ductility is the deflection corresponding to rupture strength. (*From* El Khwad M, Stetzer B, Moore, RM. Term human fetal membranes have a weak zone overlying the lower uterine pole and cervix before onset of labor. Biol Reprod. 2005;72(3)723; with permission.)

metalloproteinases (TIMPs) (1–3), apoptosis, fibulin family proteins, elastin/collagen content, collagen fiber alignment, Pyridium cross-linking and collagen microstructure.[7,8,16,24,25,29,35–46] For a more detailed review of FM strength characteristics readers are directed to our previous reviews.[6–8]

FETAL MEMBRANES HAVE A PHYSIOLOGIC WEAK ZONE

To understand the biomechanical properties of the FM, freshly obtained membranes were obtained and systematically measured and mapped over the entire surface and then correlated with local biochemical properties in term and preterm FM.[15,16,47] These studies have revealed that the FMs are not homogeneous. A focal physiologic "Weak Zone" with increased collagen remodeling and apoptosis relative to the rest of the tissue develops in the region overlying the cervix.[15,16] The spontaneous rupture tear line usually extends through the weak zone. This region of the FM was initially identified as morphologically different by Steven Bell and colleagues.[17,18] Several groups have characterized this weak zone extensively and confirmed increased extracellular matrix (ECM) remodeling, apoptosis, inflammation, and chorion thinning in this region.[19,21–23,48–52] Other processes that may contribute to the FM weakening and rupture include disorganization of collagen fiber bundles, "phenotypic switching" of mesenchymal cells from strength promoting myofibroblasts to macrophages capable of producing inflammatory cytokines, that is associated with a decrease in production of fibulin proteins in the paracervical weak zone.[43,53,54]

The amnion and chorion separate at term. Developmentally, in early pregnancy, the amnion and chorion are separate and fuse between 14 and 16 weeks of gestation. Later during parturition at term, before FM rupture, the amnion separates from choriodecidua in the physiologic paracervical weak zone as part of normal FM weakening and rupture. This appears to be a nearly universal occurrence.[34,55,56] Collagen fiber disorganization due to decorin and biglycan changes, and water absorption due to increases in hyaluronan at the amnion-chorio-decidua (CD) interface may contribute to this process.[57,58]

FMs must weaken before rupture occurs. A significant body of work suggests that the term FM must be weakened as a result of programmed biochemically mediated processes. This occurs before mechanical stresses of labor contractions begin. Preterm FM weakening and pPROM occurs when these same biochemical-mediated processes are exaggerated and occur prematurely due to infection/inflammation or when decidual bleeding-abruption occur. Preterm FMs are stronger than term FMs with a significant drop-off in rupture strength after 37 to 38 weeks' gestation.[47,59,60] It is thus clear that pPROM requires a more extensive biochemical weakening process than at term.

THE PATHWAY OF HUMAN FETAL MEMBRANE WEAKENING

There are no animal models to investigate human FM weakening and pPROM. Cell model systems cannot address tissue-level weakening. For this reason, human FM explant culture systems are used to evaluate the biomechanical properties, like rupture strength. This model system has been successfully used to explore the mechanisms of FM weakening, and also test agents that may potentially prevent the weakening. These systems can explore potential therapeutic interventions.[6–8,13–16,24,25,34–44,47,55,56,61–65]

A number of pathologic clinical processes share common pathways. Ascending bacterial infections from the maternal genital tract are widely speculated to cause pPROM; up to 55% of patients exhibit culture or polymerase chain reaction evidence of infection.[66] pPROM is associated with elevated levels of inflammatory cytokines (interleukin-1β [IL-1β], IL-6, IL-8), tumor necrosis factor-α (TNF), granulocyte-macrophage colony-stimulating factor (GM-CSF), and also with the generation of thrombin in amniotic fluid and FM.[26,67–71] There is significant crosstalk between inflammation and abruption-coagulation systems and they frequently occur together. Principal mediators of this cross talk are cytokines, thrombin, and tissue factor. Abruption and pPROM lead to increased tissue factor production and thrombin generation by the choriondecidua.[72,73] Although thrombin is a primary mediator of the coagulation cascade, it also promotes expression of MMPs and neutrophil chemo-attracting and chemo-activating chemokines precipitating pPROM-preterm birth.[25,41]

Cytokines and thrombin can weaken FM in vitro. For these reasons, TNF or IL-1β are as surrogates for infection/inflammation and, thrombin, as a surrogate for decidual bleeding/abruption, the prime drivers of pPROM.[7] Using fresh, strong FM distal from the weak zone described previously, we demonstrated that the inflammatory cytokines TNF and IL-1, and thrombin each weaken full-thickness FM explants in a concentration-dependent manner (**Fig. 2**). Furthermore, concomitant with weakening, the tissue demonstrates increased remodeling and apoptosis, which mimics that seen in the physiologic weak zone of term FM.[24,25,36,41,42] This in vitro model simulated the FM weakening process.

Cytokines and thrombin weaken FM by targeting the CD but not the amnion. Preterm birth and specifically pPROM is often precipitated by adverse stimuli such as infection and abruption/decidual bleeding. These events originate from the maternal-decidual side, we investigated whether the targets of the TNF, IL-1β, and thrombin that had been shown to cause FM weakening were in the amnion or the CD.[68,74–77] This information is important both for understanding the FM weakening

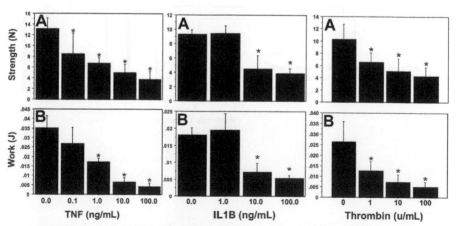

Fig. 2. Cytokine and thrombin weakening of fetal membranes (left, middle, and right). TNF, IL-1β, and thrombin each induce concentration-dependent decreases in FM strength (*A*) and work to rupture (*B*) (data as mean ± SD, *P<.01) (left and middle panels). (*From* Kumar D, Fung W, Moore RM. Proinflammatory cytokines found in amniotic fluid induce collagen remodeling, apoptosis, and biophysical weakening of cultured human fetal membranes. Biol Reprod. 2006;74(1):29–34; with permission. [Right panel] *From* Moore RM, Schatz F, Kumar D, et al. Alpha-lipoic acid inhibits thrombin-induced fetal membrane weakening in vitro. Placenta. 2010;31(10):888; with permission.)

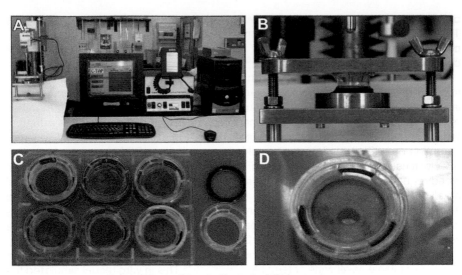

Cultured Transwell insert with attached FM fragment

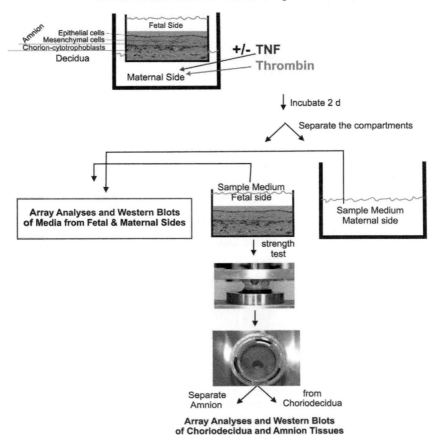

process and for identifying possible therapeutic agents for the prevention of pPROM. The amnion is the strongest component of the FM and must be significantly weakened before rupture of membranes can occur but it is unclear whether amnion was targeted directly by cytokines and thrombin.[34,47]

As the amnion is readily separated from the CD, these experiments proved relatively straightforward. TNF and IL-1 readily weaken intact FM but they do not weaken isolated amnion. When isolated CD are incubated with TNF or IL-1, the media produced readily weakens the amnion. It is thus clear that these cytokines target the CD and not the amnion.[25] Thrombin's interaction with FM components is more complicated. Thrombin can affect the isolated amnion. However, for thrombin to weaken amnion directly it needs to first traverse the chorion in significant concentration from decidual bleeding points to reach the amnion.[40,41] Using our model system as described in detail later in this article, we not only validated that thrombin (and also TNF) when applied to the maternal facing compartment causes a concentration-dependent decrease in FM strength, but also that thrombin did not pass through the FM to the amnion side.[40]

Because of the clear directionality (from maternal side toward fetal side) of the pathway of FM weakening in both, the in vivo and the in vitro studies, we modified our culture system to provide directionality.[7] The enhanced system allows one to apply test agents (eg, IL-1ß, TNF, thrombin) to either the decidual (maternal) or amniotic (fetal) side of an FM explant and follow the effect directionally through the tissue (**Fig. 3**). For this system, the semipermeable membrane in Transwell insert is removed and replaced with either intact FM or an FM component (amnion or chorion-decidua) that are held in place (like a drum skin) with an O-ring. The insert is then placed into a matching culture well and media is applied to the dish (lower) and the insert (upper). Thus, the maternal and fetal sides of the FM can be treated separately by applying test agents to the upper or lower chambers. The tissue is incubated in experimental conditions for up to 3 days at 37°C and then strength tested after incubations without any manipulation. Afterward the tissue is available for biochemical and immunohistochemical (IHC) analysis (see **Fig. 3**). With this new system we showed that both TNF and thrombin-induced FM weakening in a concentration-dependent manner when applied only to the CD side of the FM[40,61] (**Fig. 4**).

The cytokine GM-CSF appears to be critical intermediate in both the TNF and thrombin-induced FM weakening pathways. When it became known that TNF and

---

Fig. 3. The enhanced model system for testing FM strength. Top: (*A*) FM strength testing system. (*B*) Six Transwells with mounted FM in a culture dish and a Transwell without FM shown at right. (*C*) Close up of a Transwell mounted between the horizontal plates in the rupture testing equipment with plunger approaching perpendicularly. (*D*) Transwell with punctured, strength tested FM. Bottom: Schematic: Full-thickness FM fragments with CD down-mounted Transwell inserts in culture plates in medium. Thus, 2 compartments are formed (fetal, above the amnion, and maternal, below the CD). Activators (eg, TNF, thrombin) or their inhibitors can be applied to either compartment, medium is sampled after incubations and FM fragments are strength tested within the Transwell insert. Thereafter, separated amnion and CD components, and conditioned medium, are available for analysis. (*From* Kumar D, Moore RM, Nash A, et al. Decidual GM-CSF is a critical common intermediate necessary for thrombin and TNF induced in-vitro fetal membrane weakening. Placenta. 2014;35(12):1051; with permission.)

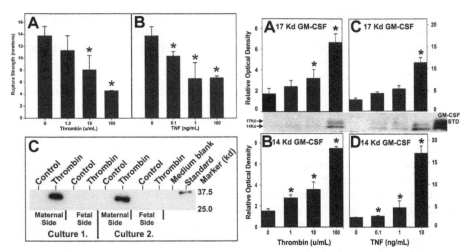

Fig. 4. Left: Validation of the enhanced model system. Unidirectional CD (maternal) compartment application of thrombin (A) or TNF (B) on cultured FM caused concentration-dependent decreases in FM rupture strength (data as mean ± SD, *P<.05). (C) Thrombin does not pass through the FM during the weakening process after application of the highest dose of Thrombin to the CD compartment. Right: Thrombin and TNF both increase GM-CSF in the CD compartment. Thrombin and TNF increase 14 KD and 17 KD GM-CSF proteins in CD medium (Thrombin: A and B; TNF: C and D). (data as mean ± SD, *P<.05). (*From* Kumar D, Moore RM, Nash A, et al. Decidual GM-CSF is a critical common intermediate necessary for thrombin and TNF induced in-vitro fetal membrane weakening. Placenta. 2014;35(12):1049–56; with permission.)

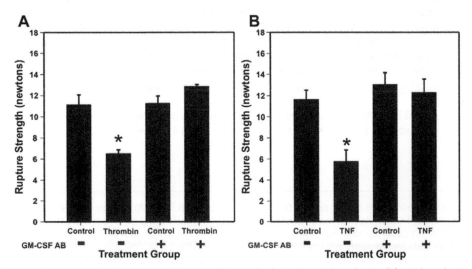

Fig. 5. GM-CSF is a critical intermediate for both thrombin (A) and TNF (B) -induced FM weakening. GM-CSF antibody inhibits thrombin and TNF-induced FM weakening. FM fragments were pre-incubated in the CD compartment with or without GM-CSF neutralizing antibody followed by (for 48 hours) with or without addition of thrombin (10 μ/mL) (A) or TNF (10 ng/mL) (B) and then strength tested (data as mean ± SD, *P<.05). (*From* Kumar D, Moore RM, Nash A, et al. Decidual GM-CSF is a critical common intermediate necessary for thrombin and TNF induced in-vitro fetal membrane weakening. Placenta. 2014;35(12):1054; with permission.)

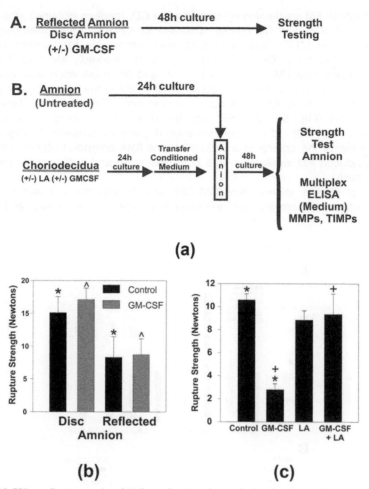

(a)

(b)   (c)

Fig. 6. GM-CSF mediates amnion (AM) weakening through the choriodecidua (CD). (a) Study Design: A. To determine if GM-CSF weakens AM alone, reflected, as well as disc AM were separately cultured ± 200 ng/mL GM-CSF for 48 hours then strength tested. B. AM was separated from CD. AM was cultured for 24 hours without additions while CD was treated with/without 100 μM LA and with/without 200 ng/mL GM-CSF for 24 hours. Media were then transferred to the washed AM cultures and incubated for an additional 48 hours. AM strength was determined and media from treatment groups were frozen for multiplex enzyme-linked immunosorbent assay (ELISA). (b) Results: Although disc AM was significantly stronger than reflected AM, GM-CSF (200 ng/mL) did not directly weaken AM from either region at doses that weakened full thickness FM. The initial target of GM-CSF in its weakening effect on FM is not the AM. (c) Results: GM-CSF (200 ng/mL) conditioned CD medium induced marked weakening in the isolated AM (*<.05). In addition, CD conditioned medium following α-lipoic acid (LA) (100 μM) co-incubation with GM-CSF (GM-CSF + LA) does not weaken isolated AM (rupture strength in Newtons [N] as m ± SD); symbols designate pairs of columns with significant differences (*, + indicate *P*<.05). (*From* Sharma A, Kumar D, Moore RM, et al. Granulocyte macrophage colony stimulating factor (GM-CSF), the critical intermediate of inflammation-induced fetal membrane weakening, primarily exerts its weakening effect on the choriodecidua rather than the amnion. Placenta. 2020;89(1):4; with permission.)

thrombin initiate FM weakening by targeting the CD, medium obtained after TNF or thrombin incubated with CD (alone), a screen for cytokines and chemokines that might induce the MMPs and other proteases responsible for weakening of the amnion was performed. GM-CSF was found to be markedly elevated. Follow-up studies revealed that FM weakening by TNF and thrombin each was associated with a concentration-dependent induction of GM-CSF in the CD compartment (see **Fig. 4**). GM-CSF neutralizing antibody blocked both TNF and thrombin-induced FM weakening (**Fig. 5**). GM-CSF was found to readily weaken full-thickness (adherent amnion-CD) FM in a concentration-dependent manner[37,40] (**Fig. 6**). GM-CSF thus meets the criteria of a critical intermediate compound for inflammation/bleeding-induced FM weakening. It is both necessary and sufficient for the weakening process.

Additional studies showed that GM-CSF also targets the CD rather than the amnion, where it increases the expression of specific proteases and inhibits

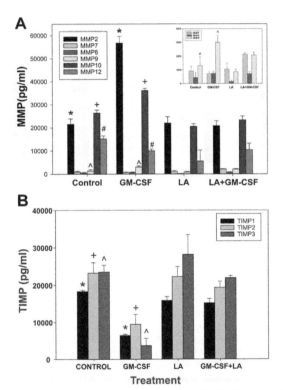

Fig. 7. GM-CSF induced MMP secretion in the choriodecidua (CD) (*A*) and reduced CD TIMP production (*B*). In addition, α-LA reversed these GM-CSF induced changes. Conditioned media (as described in **Fig. 6**) were analyzed by Multiplex ELISA for presence of MMPs (1, 2, 3, 7, 8, 9, 10, 12, and 13, BIO-RAD, multiplex) and TIMPs (1, 2, 3, and 4) MMPs 1,3,13 and TIMP4 were not detected in CD conditioned media. (data as mean ± SD). Symbols designate pairs of columns with significant differences (*P*<.05). (*From* Sharma A, Kumar D, Moore RM, et al. Granulocyte macrophage colony stimulating factor (GM-CSF), the critical intermediate of inflammation-induced fetal membrane weakening, primarily exerts its weakening effect on the choriodecidua rather than the amnion. Placenta. 2020;89(1):4; with permission.)

expression of protease inhibitors in the FM[37] (see **Fig. 6**; **Fig. 7**). Based on those findings, we concluded that GM-CSF weakens the FM by increasing net proteolytic activity that degrades the amnion ECM. GM-CSF is thus a critical intermediate compound in both TNF and thrombin-induced FM weakening pathways, making it a particularly important potential target for therapeutic intervention to prevent pPROM.

Clinical findings support a role for GM-CSF in preterm birth. FM from pregnancies complicated by chorioamnionitis, abruption, or idiopathic preterm birth versus FM from uncomplicated term normal pregnancies stain more intensely for GM-

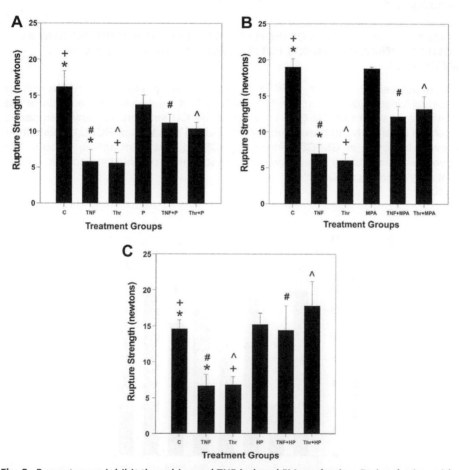

Fig. 8. Progestogens inhibit thrombin- and TNF-induced FM weakening. Preincubation with (*A*) progesterone, (*B*) MPA, or (*C*) 17a-hydroxyprogesterone for 24 hours inhibited FM weakening by either TNF or Thr applied for 48 additional hours. In all studies, all agents were applied to only the CD side of the FM. Strength testing was done at 72 hours. (data as mean ± SD). Symbols designate pairs of columns with significant differences (*A*, * and + indicate $P<.01$, and ˆ and # indicate $P<.05$; *B*, *, +, ˆ indicate $P<.01$, and # indicates $P<.02$; *C*, all of the symbols indicate $P<.01$). C, control; HP, 17a-hydroxyprogesterone; MPA, Medroxyprogesterone acetate; P, progesterone; Thr, thrombin; TNF, tumor necrosis factor α. (*From* Kumar D, Springel RM, Moore BM, et al. Progesterone inhibits in vitro fetal membrane weakening. Am J Obstet Gynecol. 2015;213(4):520.e3; with permission.)

CSF localized to decidual cells.[36,78] Further, cultured decidual cells from such complicated pregnancies when treated with TNF, IL-1, or thrombin cause a significant induction of GM-CSF.[36,78] GM-CSF chemotactic activity and granulocyte attraction were shown to be greater in PROM (premature rupture at term before labor) compared with term FM ruptured after labor onset.[68] GM-CSF presumably recruits mononuclear cells, activates monocyte conversion to macrophages, and activates macrophages resulting in protease production, eventually resulting in FM weakening. GM-CSF may not act completely alone in these latter steps. One such example is the reported requisite synergistic action between GM-CSF and TNF for monocytes to induce MMP1 and MMP9 with roles in collagen remodeling.[79]

EVALUATION OF INHIBITORS OF THE FETAL MEMBRANE WEAKENING PATHWAY AS POSSIBLE THERAPEUTIC AGENTS FOR PRETERM PREMATURE RUPTURE OF MEMBRANES

We hypothesized that for pPROM to occur due to inflammation/infection or decidual bleeding/abruption, the FM must be first weakened as the result of the downstream action of GM-CSF induced at the CD junction. For any therapeutic agent to be effective in preventing FM weakening and thus pPROM, it must either prevent induction of GM-CSF, inhibit GM-CSF downstream action, or both. We have used this strategy in our in vitro model to screen potential therapeutic agents that may prevent pPROM.[6,7]

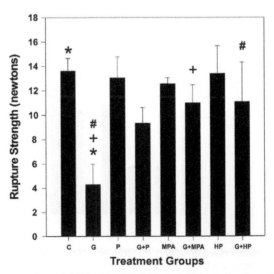

Fig. 9. Progesterone analogs inhibit GM-CSF induced FM weakening. Preincubation with progesterone, MPA or HP for 24 hr inhibited FM weakening by GM-CSF applied for 48 additional hr. All agents were applied only to the CD side of the FM. Strength testing was done at 72 h for all FM fragments (data as mean ± SD). Symbols (*, +, #) designate pairs of columns with significant differences (all $P<.01$). Definitions: C, control; G, GM-CSF; P, progesterone; MPA, medroxyprogesterone acetate; HP, 17a-hydroxyprogesterone. (*From* Kumar D, Springel RM, Moore BM, et al. Progesterone inhibits in vitro fetal membrane weakening. Am J Obstet Gynecol. 2015;213(4):520.e5; with permission.)

Progesterone and Its Analogs

The American College of Obstetricians and Gynecologist's current recommendation for prevention of recurrent preterm birth is weekly intramuscular administration of 17-α hydroxyprogesterone caproate (17-OHPC) or daily vaginal administration of progesterone for a short cervical length.[80] However, current evidence strongly suggests that these agents lack efficacy.[81] We have investigated ability of progestogens to inhibit FM weakening by TNF modeling infection/inflammation and thrombin modeling decidual bleeding-abruption. The 3 progestogens, progesterone, 17-α-hydroxyprogesterone (17-OHP; natural analog)p and medroxyprogesterone acetate (MPA), inhibit both TNF and thrombin-induced FM weakening by inhibiting both the production of GM-CSF and also downstream GM-CSF action[63] (**Figs. 8** and **9**). In contrast, the clinically used 17-OHPC inhibits FM weakening pathway only at the level of GM-CSF production but not its downstream action[39] (**Figs. 10–12**). Based on these studies, 17-OHPC would be less likely to be effective than the other progestins. As GM-CSF can be produced in other tissues outside the FM and also as the result of senescence and other processes, a progestin with effects only on GM-CSF production in FM, would clearly be less desirable.

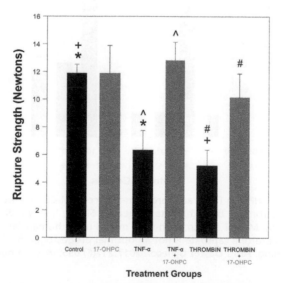

Fig. 10. 17-OHPC inhibits TNF-α and thrombin-induced FM weakening. Preincubation with 17-OHPC for 24 hours inhibited FM weakening by either TNF or thrombin applied for 48 additional hours. All agents applied only to the CD side of FM. Strength testing performed at 72 hours (data as mean ± SD). * and + indicate $P<.01$; ^ and # indicate $P<.05$. 17-OHPC, 17-alpha hydroxyprogesterone caproate. Kumar and colleagues 17-OHPC not an optimal progestogen for inhibition of fetal membrane weakening. (*From* Kumar D, Moore RM, Mercer BM. In an in-vitro model using human fetal membranes, 17-alpha hydroxyprogesterone caproate is not an optimal progestogen for inhibition of fetal membrane weakening. Am J Obstet Gynecol. 2017;217(6):695.e6; with permission.)

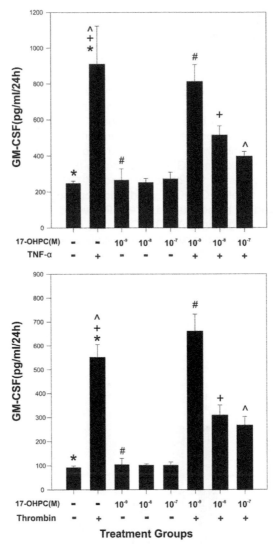

Fig. 11. Effect of 17-OHPC on TNF-α and thrombin-induced GM-CSF release on the CD side of FM (TNF: top, and thrombin: bottom) (data as mean ± SD) (*, ^, +, # indicate P<.01). (*From* Kumar D, Moore RM, Mercer BM. In an in-vitro model using human fetal membranes, 17-alpha hydroxyprogesterone caproate is not an optimal progestogen for inhibition of fetal membrane weakening. Am J Obstet Gynecol. 2017;217(6):695.e8; with permission.)

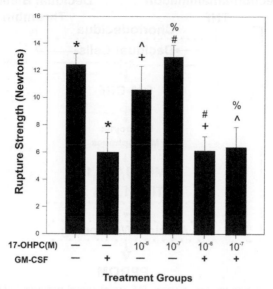

Fig. 12. 17-OHPC fails to inhibit GM-CSF-induced FM weakening. Preincubation with 17-OHPC for 24 hours failed to inhibit FM weakening by GM-CSF (200 ng/mL) applied for 48 additional hours. All agents applied only to the CD side of FM. Strength testing was performed at 72 hours (*, #, % indicate $P<.01$, and + and ^ indicate $P<.05$). (*From* Kumar D, Moore RM, Mercer BM. In an in-vitro model using human fetal membranes, 17-alpha hydroxyprogesterone caproate is not an optimal progestogen for inhibition of fetal membrane weakening. Am J Obstet Gynecol. 2017;217(6):695.e9; with permission.)

NONPROGESTIN AGENTS

Studies done in vitro and in nonpregnant humans suggest that α-lipoic acid (LA) may be a useful agent for prevention of pPROM. LA is a natural dietary supplement with metal chelation, antioxidant and nuclear factor–κB inhibitory properties. It is used commonly for prophylaxis to prevent diabetic neuropathy.[82] Toxicity studies in rodent models have been promising and it is being trialed as a therapeutic agent for a variety of disorders (clinicaltrials.gov).[83] In our model system, LA blocks both TNF and thrombin-induced intact FM weakening, and concomitant collagen remodeling as evidenced by inhibition of MMP9, MMP3, and PGE2.[42,44] LA blocks TNF and thrombin-induced FM weakening at 2 points, GM-CSF production and its downstream action.[37,38] LA therefore would theoretically be a potential candidate to prevent spontaneous preterm birth. A trial of LA to prevent pPROM in pregnant women at risk awaits more definitive information on its mechanism of action in preventing FM weakening, in addition to safety data.

In addition to LA, vitamin C has been trialed and proven unable to prevent FM weakening or to clinically prevent preterm birth.[64,84] The Lappas Group has also reported that a number of other anti-inflammatory dietary agents have the potential to prevent prematurity.[85,86] The anti-inflammatory agent N-acetylcysteine has been used in a small double-blind clinical trial showing efficacy in preventing preterm birth in women at risk for preterm birth.[87] These agents warrant examination in preventing FM weakening and pPROM but have not been screened for their effect on inflammation/bleeding-induced FM weakening.

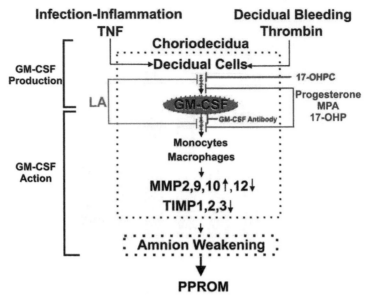

Fig. 13. Proposed mechanism for human FM weakening pathways. (1) TNF (modeling inflammation) and thrombin (modeling decidual bleeding/abruption) weaken FM in vitro. (2) TNF and thrombin induce CD production of the critical intermediate GM-CSF by decidual stromal cells. GM-CSF neutralizing antibody blocks both TNF and thrombin-induced weakening. (3) We have hypothesized that GM-CSF recruits and activates mononuclear cells, then activates macrophages that produce proteases to cause FM weakening. MMPs 2, 9, 10 increase and TIMPs 1 to 3 decrease when CD is stimulated with GM-CSF. (4) Progestogens (P4, MPA, and 17-OHP) inhibit both GM-CSF production and GM-CSF action, but 17-OHPC only inhibits GM-CSF production (not GM-CSF action) and thus may be less efficacious in clinical use than other agents. (5) LA inhibits both GM-CSF production by TNF/thrombin and also GM-CSF downstream weakening activity. P4, progesterone; MPA, medroxyprogesterone acetate; 17-OHP, 17α-Hydroxy-progesterone. (*From* Sharma A, Kumar D, Moore RM, et al. Granulocyte macrophage colony stimulating factor (GM-CSF), the critical intermediate of inflammation-induced fetal membrane weakening, primarily exerts its weakening effect on the choriodecidua rather than the amnion. Placenta. 2020;89(1):5; with permission.)

SUMMARY

The line of work reviewed here uses an in vitro model system that combines biochemical/histologic with mechanical/engineering approaches. The model highlights potential mechanistic reasons for lack of efficacy of currently clinically used agents to prevent preterm birth. Likewise, it can be used to screen agents with potential for preventing pPROM and preterm birth. The cumulative results of these studies are illustrated in **Fig. 13**. These studies provide a unique perspective and information about the physiology of FM weakening and rupture.

DISCLOSURE

The authors have nothing to disclose.

CLINICS CARE POINTS

- Inflammatory agents induce FM weakening leading to membrane rupture by acting through GM-CSF generated locally in the decidua. Thus, potential therapeutic agents to prevent preterm births associated with inflammation-induced

FM weakening and pPROM should ideally block both the production and the downstream action of GM-CSF in the FM.

- Although high doses of most Progesterone analogs inhibit both inflammation-induced GM-CSF production and its downstream action in FM explants, the clinically used 17α-Hydroxy-progesterone caproate only inhibits inflammation-induced GM-CSF production, and not GM-CSF downstream action. This makes it potentially less effective in preventing pPROM.
- Alpha-lipoic acid, an over-the-counter anti-oxidant, inhibits both inflammation-induced GM-CSF production and its downstream action in FM explants. If vetted properly for use in pregnant women, it might prove clinically useful to prevent pPROM.
- There are no animal models for pPROM, so the studies reviewed here were done in explants of full thickness human FM. The concentrations of possible therapeutic agents used in these studies may not be attainable in vivo.

REFERENCES

1. Beck S, Wojdyla D, Say L, et al. The worldwide incidence of preterm birth: a systematic review of maternal mortality and morbidity. Bull World Health Organ 2010; 88(1):31–8.
2. Blencowe H, Krasevec J, de Onis M, et al. National, regional, and worldwide estimates of low birthweight in 2015, with trends from 2000: a systematic analysis. Lancet Glob Health 2019;7(7):e849–60.
3. Parry S, Strauss JF 3rd. Premature rupture of the fetal membranes. N Engl J Med 1998;338(10):663–70.
4. Mercer BM. Preterm premature rupture of the membranes. Obstet Gynecol 2003; 101(1):178–93.
5. Mercer BM. Preterm premature rupture of the membranes: current approaches to evaluation and management. Obstet Gynecol Clin North Am 2005;32(3):411–28.
6. Menon R, Moore JJ. Fetal membranes, not a mere appendage of the placenta, but a critical part of the fetal-maternal interface controlling parturition. Obstet Gynecol Clin North Am 2020;47(1):147–62.
7. Kumar D, Moore RM, Mercer BM, et al. The physiology of fetal membrane weakening and rupture: Insights gained from the determination of physical properties revisited. Placenta 2016;42:59–73.
8. Moore RM, Mansour JM, Redline RW, et al. The physiology of fetal membrane rupture: insight gained from the determination of physical properties. Placenta 2006;27(11–12):1037–51.
9. Mercer BM, Goldenberg RL, Moawad AH, et al. The preterm prediction study: effect of gestational age and cause of preterm birth on subsequent obstetric outcome. National Institute of Child Health and Human Development Maternal-Fetal Medicine Units Network. Am J Obstet Gynecol 1999;181(5 Pt 1):1216–21.
10. Mercer BM. Preterm premature rupture of the membranes: diagnosis and management. Clin Perinatol 2004;31(4):765–82, vi.
11. Lockwood CJ, Toti P, Arcuri F, et al. Mechanisms of abruption-induced premature rupture of the fetal membranes: thrombin-enhanced interleukin-8 expression in term decidua. Am J Pathol 2005;167(5):1443–9.
12. Toppozada MK, Sallam NA, Gaafar AA, et al. Role of repeated stretching in the mechanism of timely rupture of the membranes. Am J Obstet Gynecol 1970; 108(2):243–9.

13. Pandey V, Jaremko K, Moore RM, et al. The force required to rupture fetal membranes paradoxically increases with acute in vitro repeated stretching. Am J Obstet Gynecol 2007;196(2):165.e1-7.
14. Joyce EM, Diaz P, Tamarkin S, et al. In-vivo stretch of term human fetal membranes. Placenta 2016;38:57–66.
15. El Khwad M, Stetzer B, Moore RM, et al. Term human fetal membranes have a weak zone overlying the lower uterine pole and cervix before onset of labor. Biol Reprod 2005;72(3):720–6.
16. El Khwad M, Pandey V, Stetzer B, et al. Fetal membranes from term vaginal deliveries have a zone of weakness exhibiting characteristics of apoptosis and remodeling. J Soc Gynecol Investig 2006;13(3):191–5.
17. Malak TM, Bell SC. Structural characteristics of term human fetal membranes: a novel zone of extreme morphological alteration within the rupture site. Br J Obstet Gynaecol 1994;101(5):375–86.
18. McLaren J, Malak TM, Bell SC. Structural characteristics of term human fetal membranes prior to labour: identification of an area of altered morphology overlying the cervix. Hum Reprod 1999;14(1):237–41.
19. McLaren J, Taylor DJ, Bell SC. Increased concentration of pro-matrix metalloproteinase 9 in term fetal membranes overlying the cervix before labor: implications for membrane remodeling and rupture. Am J Obstet Gynecol 2000;182(2): 409–16.
20. McParland PC, Taylor DJ, Bell SC. Myofibroblast differentiation in the connective tissues of the amnion and chorion of term human fetal membranes-implications for fetal membrane rupture and labour. Placenta 2000;21(1):44–53.
21. McParland PC, Taylor DJ, Bell SC. Mapping of zones of altered morphology and chorionic connective tissue cellular phenotype in human fetal membranes (amniochorion and decidua) overlying the lower uterine pole and cervix before labor at term. Am J Obstet Gynecol 2003;189(5):1481–8.
22. Chai M, Barker G, Menon R, et al. Increased oxidative stress in human fetal membranes overlying the cervix from term non-labouring and post labour deliveries. Placenta 2012;33(8):604–10.
23. Reti NG, Lappas M, Riley C, et al. Why do membranes rupture at term? Evidence of increased cellular apoptosis in the supracervical fetal membranes. Am J Obstet Gynecol 2007;196(5):021.
24. Kumar D, Fung W, Moore RM, et al. Proinflammatory cytokines found in amniotic fluid induce collagen remodeling, apoptosis, and biophysical weakening of cultured human fetal membranes. Biol Reprod 2006;74(1):29–34.
25. Kumar D, Schatz F, Moore RM, et al. The effects of thrombin and cytokines upon the biomechanics and remodeling of isolated amnion membrane, in vitro. Placenta 2011;32(3):206–13.
26. Kacerovsky M, Celec P, Vlkova B, et al. Amniotic fluid protein profiles of intraamniotic inflammatory response to Ureaplasma spp. and other bacteria. PLoS One 2013;8(3):e60399.
27. Fortunato SJ, Menon R, Lombardi SJ. Role of tumor necrosis factor-alpha in the premature rupture of membranes and preterm labor pathways. Am J Obstet Gynecol 2002;187(5):1159–62.
28. Fortunato SJ, Menon R. IL-1 beta is a better inducer of apoptosis in human fetal membranes than IL-6. Placenta 2003;24(10):922–8.
29. Moore RM, Silver RJ, Moore JJ. Physiological apoptotic agents have different effects upon human amnion epithelial and mesenchymal cells. Placenta 2003; 24(2–3):173–80.

30. Moore RM, Lundgren DW, Silver RJ, et al. Lactosylceramide-induced apoptosis in primary amnion cells and amnion-derived WISH cells. J Soc Gynecol Investig 2002;9(5):282–9.
31. Zaga V, Estrada-Gutierrez G, Beltran-Montoya J, et al. Secretions of interleukin-1beta and tumor necrosis factor alpha by whole fetal membranes depend on initial interactions of amnion or choriodecidua with lipopolysaccharides or group B streptococci. Biol Reprod 2004;71(4):1296–302.
32. Fortunato SJ, Menon R, Bryant C, et al. Programmed cell death (apoptosis) as a possible pathway to metalloproteinase activation and fetal membrane degradation in premature rupture of membranes. Am J Obstet Gynecol 2000;182(6):1468–76.
33. McLaren J, Taylor DJ, Bell SC. Increased incidence of apoptosis in non-labour-affected cytotrophoblast cells in term fetal membranes overlying the cervix. Hum Reprod 1999;14(11):2895–900.
34. Arikat S, Novince RW, Mercer BM, et al. Separation of amnion from choriodecidua is an integral event to the rupture of normal term fetal membranes and constitutes a significant component of the work required. Am J Obstet Gynecol 2006;194(1):211–7.
35. Burzle W, Mazza E, Moore JJ. About puncture testing applied for mechanical characterization of fetal membranes. J Biomech Eng 2014;136(11).
36. Sinkey RG, Guzeloglu-Kayisli O, Arlier S, et al. Thrombin-induced decidual colony-stimulating factor-2 promotes abruption-related preterm birth by weakening fetal membranes. Am J Pathol 2020;190(2):388–99.
37. Sharma A, Kumar D, Moore RM, et al. Granulocyte macrophage colony stimulating factor (GM-CSF), the critical intermediate of inflammation-induced fetal membrane weakening, primarily exerts its weakening effect on the choriodecidua rather than the amnion. Placenta 2020;89:1–7.
38. Kumar D, Moore RM, Sharma A, et al. In an in-vitro model using human fetal membranes, alpha-lipoic acid inhibits inflammation induced fetal membrane weakening. Placenta 2018;68:9–14.
39. Kumar D, Moore RM, Mercer BM, et al. In an in-vitro model using human fetal membranes, 17-alpha hydroxyprogesterone caproate is not an optimal progestogen for inhibition of fetal membrane weakening. Am J Obstet Gynecol 2017;217(6):695.e1-14.
40. Kumar D, Moore RM, Nash A, et al. Decidual GM-CSF is a critical common intermediate necessary for thrombin and TNF induced in-vitro fetal membrane weakening. Placenta 2014;35(12):1049–56.
41. Puthiyachirakkal M, Lemerand K, Kumar D, et al. Thrombin weakens the amnion extracellular matrix (ECM) directly rather than through protease activated receptors. Placenta 2013;34(10):924–31.
42. Moore RM, Schatz F, Kumar D, et al. Alpha-lipoic acid inhibits thrombin-induced fetal membrane weakening in vitro. Placenta 2010;31(10):886–92.
43. Moore RM, Redline RW, Kumar D, et al. Differential expression of fibulin family proteins in the para-cervical weak zone and other areas of human fetal membranes. Placenta 2009;30(4):335–41.
44. Moore RM, Novak JB, Kumar D, et al. Alpha-lipoic acid inhibits tumor necrosis factor-induced remodeling and weakening of human fetal membranes. Biol Reprod 2009;80(4):781–7.
45. Buerzle W, Haller CM, Jabareen M, et al. Multiaxial mechanical behavior of human fetal membranes and its relationship to microstructure. Biomech Model Mechanobiol 2013;12(4):747–62.

46. Jabareen M, Mallik AS, Bilic G, et al. Relation between mechanical properties and microstructure of human fetal membranes: an attempt towards a quantitative analysis. Eur J Obstet Gynecol Reprod Biol 2009;144(Suppl 1):S134–41.
47. Rangaswamy N, Abdelrahim A, Moore RM, et al. [Biomechanical characteristics of human fetal membranes. Preterm fetal membranes are stronger than term fetal membranes]. Gynecol Obstet Fertil 2011;39(6):373–7.
48. Premyslova M, Li W, Alfaidy N, et al. Differential expression and regulation of microsomal prostaglandin E(2) synthase in human fetal membranes and placenta with infection and in cultured trophoblast cells. J Clin Endocrinol Metab 2003; 88(12):6040–7.
49. McParland PC, Bell SC, Pringle JH, et al. Regional and cellular localization of osteonectin/SPARC expression in connective tissue and cytotrophoblastic layers of human fetal membranes at term. Mol Hum Reprod 2001;7(5):463–74.
50. McLaren J, Taylor DJ, Bell SC. Prostaglandin E(2)-dependent production of latent matrix metalloproteinase-9 in cultures of human fetal membranes. Mol Hum Reprod 2000;6(11):1033–40.
51. Lappas M, Odumetse TL, Riley C, et al. Pre-labour fetal membranes overlying the cervix display alterations in inflammation and NF-kappaB signalling pathways. Placenta 2008;29(12):995–1002.
52. Fortner KB, Grotegut CA, Ransom CE, et al. Bacteria localization and chorion thinning among preterm premature rupture of membranes. PLoS One 2014; 9(1):e83338.
53. Kim SS, Romero R, Kim JS, et al. Coexpression of myofibroblast and macrophage markers: novel evidence for an in vivo plasticity of chorioamniotic mesodermal cells of the human placenta. Lab Invest 2008;88(4):365–74.
54. Connon CJ, Nakamura T, Hopkinson A, et al. The biomechanics of amnion rupture: an X-ray diffraction study. PLoS One 2007;2(11):e1147.
55. Strohl A, Kumar D, Novince R, et al. Decreased adherence and spontaneous separation of fetal membrane layers–amnion and choriodecidua–a possible part of the normal weakening process. Placenta 2010;31(1):18–24.
56. Kumar D, Novince R, Strohl A, et al. A new methodology to measure strength of adherence of the fetal membrane components, amnion and the choriodecidua. Placenta 2009;30(6):560–3.
57. Meinert M, Malmström A, Tufvesson E, et al. Labour induces increased concentrations of biglycan and hyaluronan in human fetal membranes. Placenta 2007; 28(5–6):482–6.
58. Meinert M, Eriksen GV, Petersen AC, et al. Proteoglycans and hyaluronan in human fetal membranes. Am J Obstet Gynecol 2001;184(4):679–85.
59. Pressman EK, Cavanaugh JL, Woods JR. Physical properties of the chorioamnion throughout gestation. Am J Obstet Gynecol 2002;187(3):672–5.
60. Chua WK, Oyen ML. Do we know the strength of the chorioamnion? A critical review and analysis. Eur J Obstet Gynecol Reprod Biol 2009;144(Suppl 1): S128–33.
61. Kumar D, Moore RM, Mercer BM, et al. In an in-vitro model using human fetal membranes, 17-α hydroxyprogesterone caproate is not an optimal progestogen for inhibition of fetal membrane weakening. Am J Obstet Gynecol 2017;217(6): 695.e1-14.
62. Kumar D MR, Springel E, Mercer BM, et al. Activated dendritic cells cause human amnion weakening with UPA/Serpin E1 changes that are inhibited by progesterone receptor agonists. Reproductive Sciences (March); 2016.

63. Kumar D, Springel E, Moore RM, et al. Progesterone inhibits in vitro fetal membrane weakening. Am J Obstet Gynecol 2015;213(4):520.e1-9.
64. Mercer BM, Abdelrahim A, Moore RM, et al. The impact of vitamin C supplementation in pregnancy and in vitro upon fetal membrane strength and remodeling. Reprod Sci 2010;17(7):685–95.
65. Joyce EM, Moore JJ, Sacks MS. Biomechanics of the fetal membrane prior to mechanical failure: review and implications. Eur J Obstet Gynecol Reprod Biol 2009; 144(Suppl 1):S121–7.
66. Jones HE, Harris KA, Azizia M, et al. Differing prevalence and diversity of bacterial species in fetal membranes from very preterm and term labor. PLoS One 2009;4(12):e8205.
67. Kacerovsky M, Cobo T, Andrys C, et al. The fetal inflammatory response in subgroups of women with preterm prelabor rupture of the membranes. J Matern Fetal Neonatal Med 2013;26(8):795–801.
68. Gomez-Lopez N, Hernandez-Santiago S, Lobb AP, et al. Normal and premature rupture of fetal membranes at term delivery differ in regional chemotactic activity and related chemokine/cytokine production. Reprod Sci 2013;20(3): 276–84.
69. Menon R. Spontaneous preterm birth, a clinical dilemma: etiologic, pathophysiologic and genetic heterogeneities and racial disparity. Acta Obstet Gynecol Scand 2008;87(6):590–600.
70. Keelan JA, Blumenstein M, Helliwell RJ, et al. Cytokines, prostaglandins and parturition–a review. Placenta 2003;24(46).
71. Rosen T, Kuczynski E, O'Neill LM, et al. Plasma levels of thrombin-antithrombin complexes predict preterm premature rupture of the fetal membranes. J Matern Fetal Med 2001;10(5):297–300.
72. Salafia CM, Lopez-Zeno JA, Sherer DM, et al. Histologic evidence of old intrauterine bleeding is more frequent in prematurity. Am J Obstet Gynecol 1995;173(4): 1065–70.
73. Erez O, Espinoza J, Chaiworapongsa T, et al. A link between a hemostatic disorder and preterm PROM: a role for tissue factor and tissue factor pathway inhibitor. J Matern Fetal Neonatal Med 2008;21(10):732–44.
74. Gomez-Lopez N, Vadillo-Perez L, Hernandez-Carbajal A, et al. Specific inflammatory microenvironments in the zones of the fetal membranes at term delivery. Am J Obstet Gynecol 2011;205(3):235.e15-24.
75. Gomez-Lopez N, Laresgoiti-Servitje E, Olson DM, et al. The role of chemokines in term and premature rupture of the fetal membranes: a review. Biol Reprod 2010; 82(5):809–14.
76. Christiaens I, Zaragoza DB, Guilbert L, et al. Inflammatory processes in preterm and term parturition. J Reprod Immunol 2008;79(1):50–7.
77. Menon R, Swan KF, Lyden TW, et al. Expression of inflammatory cytokines (interleukin-1 beta and interleukin-6) in amniochorionic membranes. Am J Obstet Gynecol 1995;172(2 Pt 1):493–500.
78. Arcuri F, Toti P, Buchwalder L, et al. Mechanisms of leukocyte accumulation and activation in chorioamnionitis: interleukin 1 beta and tumor necrosis factor alpha enhance colony stimulating factor 2 expression in term decidua. Reprod Sci 2009;16(5):453–61.
79. Zhang Y, McCluskey K, Fujii K, et al. Differential regulation of monocyte matrix metalloproteinase and TIMP-1 production by TNF-alpha, granulocyte-macrophage CSF, and IL-1 beta through prostaglandin-dependent and -independent mechanisms. J Immunol 1998;161(6):3071–6.

80. Practice bulletin no. 130: prediction and prevention of preterm birth. Obstet Gynecol 2012;120(4):964–73.
81. Blackwell SC, Gyamfi-Bannerman C, Biggio JR Jr, et al. 17-OHPC to Prevent Recurrent Preterm Birth in Singleton Gestations (PROLONG Study): A Multicenter, International, Randomized Double-Blind Trial. Am J Perinatol 2020; 37(2):127–36.
82. Shay KP, Moreau RF, Smith EJ, et al. Alpha-lipoic acid as a dietary supplement: molecular mechanisms and therapeutic potential. Biochim Biophys Acta 2009; 1790(10):1149–60.
83. Sugimura Y, Murase T, Kobayashi K, et al. Alpha-lipoic acid reduces congenital malformations in the offspring of diabetic mice. Diabetes Metab Res Rev 2009; 25(3):287–94.
84. Swaney P, Thorp J, Allen I. Vitamin C supplementation in pregnancy–does it decrease rates of preterm birth? A systematic review. Am J Perinatol 2014; 31(2):91–8.
85. Wijesuriya YK, Lappas M. Potent anti-inflammatory effects of honokiol in human fetal membranes and myometrium. Phytomedicine 2018;49:11–22.
86. Morwood CJ, Lappas M. The citrus flavone nobiletin reduces pro-inflammatory and pro-labour mediators in fetal membranes and myometrium: implications for preterm birth. PLoS One 2014;9(9):e108390.
87. Shahin AY, Hassanin IMA, Ismail AM, et al. Effect of oral N-acetyl cysteine on recurrent preterm labor following treatment for bacterial vaginosis. Int J Gynecol Obstet 2009;104(1):44–8.

The Short Cervix
A Critical Analysis of Diagnosis and Treatment

Eboni O. Jones, MD, Zi-Qi Liew, MD, Orion A. Rust, MD*

KEYWORDS

- Short cervix • Ultrasound • Cerclage • Progesterone

KEY POINTS

- A short cervix in the second trimester is a significant risk factor for adverse perinatal outcome and the pathophysiology is complex and multifactorial.
- Biomarkers have been developed in an effort to predict preterm birth.
- Inflammation and/or infection are strongly associated with a short cervix, spontaneous preterm birth, and preterm prelabor rupture of the membranes.
- A short cervix can be treated surgically with cerclage placement or medically with progesterone.
- Treatment protocols for singleton and multiple gestation differ considerably.

BACKGROUND

Parturition in humans usually occurs at or after 37 weeks gestation. When it occurs, the cervix undergoes a remarkable transformation from a relatively rigid structure that maintains the fetus in-utero, and then transforming into a distensible conduit through which birth takes place. Preterm parturition can be divided into 2 broad categories: spontaneous preterm birth (sPTB) with or without preterm prelabor rupture of the membranes (PPROM) and indicated preterm birth.[1] Spontaneous PTB/PPROM is a leading cause of perinatal mortality in the United States. The preterm birth rate peaked in 2004 with more than 300,000 singleton liveborn deliveries between 20 and 36 weeks gestation and was associated with 75% of all neonatal morbidity and mortality.[2] Spontaneous PTB/PPROM accounts for approximately 70% of all preterm births.[3] The cost of treatment for about 12% infants born before 37 weeks is responsible for over half of the 10 billion dollar total cost for all neonates[4] (**Table 1**). The pathophysiology of sPTB/PPROM is complex and multifactorial.[5] These diverse physiologic processes all lead to the common final parturition pathway, which is anatomically manifest by cervical dilation and effacement.[6] These anatomic changes

Department of Obstetrics and Gynecology, Lehigh Valley Health Network, 707 Hamilton Blvd, 8th Floor, Allentown, PA 18101, USA
* Corresponding author. Maternal-Fetal Medicine, 3900 Hamilton Boulevard, Suite 201, Allentown, PA 18103.
E-mail address: p8570@lvh.com

Obstet Gynecol Clin N Am 47 (2020) 545–567
https://doi.org/10.1016/j.ogc.2020.08.002
0889-8545/20/© 2020 Elsevier Inc. All rights reserved.

obgyn.theclinics.com

Table 1 Population risks	
Pregnant population (%)	
Term parturition	88
Preterm parturition	12
Preterm population (%)	
Indicated preterm birth	30
Spontaneous preterm birth	70
Cervical length screening population (%)	
Normal cervical length	98
Short cervix	2
Short cervix population (%)	
Mild or no morbidity	78
Severe morbidity or perinatal death	22

Data from Refs[1,2,6,74]

can be documented by digital examination or ultrasound.[7] Digital examination generally assesses the external cervix, whereas ultrasound can evaluate the entire cervix, including the internal os where the subtle anatomic findings of the physiologic change can first be appreciated. When these changes occur between 25 and 36 weeks this process is usually labeled as preterm labor and between 16 to 24 weeks it is labeled as cervical insufficiency. Regardless of timing or label, the process and the pathophysiology are a continuum.[8] The female cervix does not exceed a length of 6 cm and the 10th percentile for length in the pregnant population has been established at 2.5 cm.[9] Thus, a cervical length less than 2.5 cm in the second trimester is generally accepted to be a short cervix.[10] Cervical insufficiency can be diagnosed based on history (1 or more second-trimester losses with painless cervical dilation and no other cause), physical examination (painless cervical dilation in the second trimester), or by ultrasound (short cervix <2.5 cm at 16–24 weeks).[11] History alone is inadequate to make the diagnosis of cervical insufficiency, and physical diagnosis by digital pelvic examination often is a late finding in the process.[7,12] Thus, a short cervix diagnosed by ultrasound has been identified as the single most significant risk factor for sPTB/PPROM.[13] Transvaginal assessment of cervical length is the most accurate means of measurement and most reliably accomplished in the second trimester between 16 and 24 weeks gestational age.[14,15]

PATHOPHYSIOLOGY OF A SHORT CERVIX

When a patient is diagnosed with a short cervix and at risk of sPTB/PPROM, the provider should consider the pathophysiologic changes that may be affecting or occurring within the cervix. Intrinsic and extrinsic forces on the uterus can result in cervical change. Dynamic changes of the cervix, such as dilation of the internal os, prolapse of the fetal membranes into the endocervical canal, and shortening of the distal cervix can be documented on ultrasound. These changes can be elicited by extrinsic forces, such as external abdominal pressure and Valsalva or intrinsic forces, such as spontaneous or induced uterine contractions. Regardless of their origin, the changes that lead to a short cervix occur in a predictable and progressive fashion over time. Initially, the fetal membranes and endocervical canal have a near perpendicular relationship and the cervical length is measured from external to internal os. When these changes take place they begin at the internal os with widening of the proximal cervix and membranes descending into the cervical canal creating a funnel-shape. At this time, the cervical length is measured from this distal apex to the external os. Progression leads to the funnel apex reaching the external os and these changes cannot be appreciated on pelvic examination until the distal cervix widens with dilation and effacement[5] (**Fig. 1**). The cause for cervical shortening can rarely be narrowed down to 1 cause. The origin is multifactorial, involving biochemical, physical, infectious, and social stressors.

The cervix is made up of a complex connective tissue matrix, which is composed of collagen, glycosaminoglycans, proteoglycans, and elastin. When preparing for parturition, the cervix remodels and the collagen fibers disperse and crosslinks are disrupted leading to tissue laxity. Matrix metalloproteinases (MMPs) are released, which degrade collagen crosslinks and proteoglycan interactions. Decreased levels of tissue inhibitors of MMPs have also been implicated in cervical shortening and sPTB/PPROM. Placental abruption or the presence of blood is associated with PPROM. Blood can initiate a cascade of clotting factors resulting in thrombin release. Thrombin generates MMP expression, which then can initiate a cascade leading to cervical dilation, contractions, or rupture of membranes.[16]

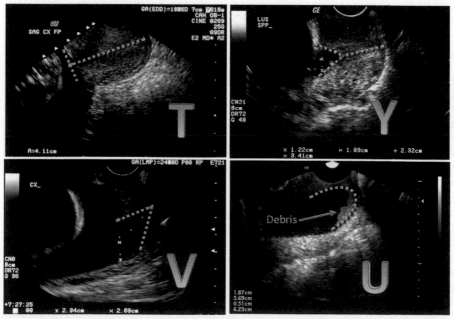

Fig. 1. Transvaginal ultrasound imaging demonstrating the progressive stages in the development of a short cervix: Upper left image shows a normal cervical length and T-shape relationship between the fetal membranes and the closed endocervical canal; Upper right image shows the Y-shape appearance of a cervical funnel characterized by dilation of the internal os, prolapse of the membranes into the endocervical canal, and shortening of the distal cervical length; Lower left image shows V-shape widening and deepening of the funnel into the endocervix with the apex approaching the external os; Lower right image shows U-shape funnel caused by further widening and deepening of membrane prolapse with dilation of the external and the finding of intraamniotic debris appearing as an echogenic inflammatory biofilm in the most dependent portion of the fetal membranes.

Maternal and fetal stressors, such as disease or deficiency can activate the hypothalamic-pituitary-adrenal axis, which has been shown to be associated with cervical shortening and subsequent preterm delivery. Increased stress is associated with increased cortisol release, which in the utero-placental environment stimulates the release of corticotropin-releasing hormone (CRH), which in turn increases prostaglandin production. Prostaglandins induce the release of placental CRH, which further contributes to the feedforward loop.[17] Prostaglandins induce the release of MMPs that can cause cervical effacement and softening. Prostaglandins directly activate uterine contractions.[18,19]

There can also be physical qualities that affect the cervix or the amniotic membranes. Any form of uterine or amniotic sac distention, such as multifetal gestation or polyhydramnios, can provoke contractions. Preexisting conditions, including maternal collagen deficiencies or connective tissue syndromes can predispose patients to having cervical insufficiency. Surgical trauma from gynecologic procedures, such as cervical excision procedures and mechanical dilation of cervix for the diagnosis and treatment of uterine pathology may have an impact on its physical properties altering the intrinsic structure of the cervix. In addition, obstetric procedures, including elective and spontaneous abortion, operative vaginal delivery, cervical laceration, and procedures to arrest obstetric hemorrhage can be associated with damage to the cervical stroma.[10] Any of these events may allow the pathophysiologic processes of preterm parturition by altering its structural properties predisposing it to cervical shortening leading to sPTB or PPROM.

SHORT CERVIX AND OTHER BIOMARKERS

Biomarkers are a means of identifying a measurable substance in an individual that predicts a phenomenon. In pregnant women, biomarkers for an increased risk of sPTB/PPROM include fetal fibronectin (FFN) and cervical length. Despite being asymptomatic, approximately 24% of women with a short cervical length will suffer PPROM, which may occur many weeks after identification.[6] Primigravid women with a cervical length of less than 2.5 cm and a positive FFN have a 1 in 6 chance of PPROM. The risk is even higher (1 in 4) for multiparous women with a similar history.[20] In addition, patients with PPROM and a shorter cervical length have been shown to have a shorter latency period to delivery.[21] FFN is a glycoprotein that is synthesized by the trophoblast and is found in the extracellular matrix of the decidua basalis adjacent to the fetal membranes. Assays of vaginal fluid for FFN have shown it to be reliably present after 20 weeks. FFN increases when there is disruption of the decidua-fetal membrane interface and serves as a biomarker for sPTB/PPROM.[22] Rigorous investigation of FFN alone and in combination with cervical length measurement determined the positive predictive value was insufficient to recommend routine screening in a low-risk population. The absence of FFN had high negative predictive value for sPTB/PPROM for 14 days after the test. Using FFN in this fashion has the potential for significant time and cost.[23] FFN has been used between 16 and 24 weeks to identify individuals at increased risk of adverse outcome with a short cervix regardless of cerclage. This information is helpful in counseling patients with respect to prognosis.[24]

Another biomarker is the presence of amniotic fluid sludge, debris, or biofilm. On sonographic imaging, echogenic collections can be seen within the amniotic sac often proximate to the cervix. This debris has been shown to be composed of fetal skin cells, vernix, leukocytes, red blood cells, and/or bacteria, and typically collects in the most dependent portions of funneled or prolapsed membranes (see **Fig. 1**, U). This finding has been reported to be associated with adverse perinatal outcome, from sPTB/

PPROM, microbial invasion of the amniotic cavity, and histologic chorioamnionitis when discovered in otherwise asymptomatic high-risk pregnancies who were being followed with serial transvaginal cervical length. The combination of this debris with a short cervix increased the risk by 10- to 15-fold over the baseline high-risk population with a normal cervical length.[25] Similar findings have been noted in twin pregnancies.[26]

There have been many studies of additional biomarker assays, including genomic, proteomic, metabolomic, and various other intermediaries of the complex preterm parturition pathways with a varying degree of results. Recently, multiple small clinical studies with results pooled in a meta-analysis have shown a qualitative assay of vaginal secretions for the glycoprotein, placental alpha macroglobulin-1, with a significant degree of sensitivity (66%) and specificity (96%) to predict sPTB within 7 days.[27] Although these results seem promising, any recommendations should await the scrutiny of larger clinical trials. In addition, as we unravel the complex pathophysiology of the short cervix, sPTB/PPROM, and parturition in general; further understanding may require the application of more advanced techniques, such as machine learning or other forms of artificial intelligence, which are emerging modalities of analysis.[28]

INFECTION AND INFLAMMATION

Infection and inflammation have frequently been shown to be associated with cervical shortening. Organisms can gain access to intrauterine tissue by an ascending infection from the vaginal microbiota, transplacental transfer from the maternal blood stream, or by way of the fallopian tubes from the peritoneal cavity. Bacteria can directly cause clinical or subclinical infection, causing a cascade of cytokines and inflammatory processes that cause prostaglandin formation and result in cervical softening, or cause uterine irritability. Bacteria can also produce toxins that can provoke the same process.[29] However, a short cervix can also be a predisposing factor for microbial invasion. Patients with a cervical length of less than 15 mm were associated with higher rate of microbial invasion (defined as a positive amniotic fluid culture) than those who had a cervical length of $\geq$30 mm.[30] Thus, a short cervix can increase the chance of infection, but an infection can also increase the occurrence of a short cervix. Organisms recovered from the amniotic fluid of pregnant women associated with an increased frequency of sPTB/PPROM include *Ureaplasma urealyticum* (most common), *Mycoplasma hominis, Fusobacterium, Neisseria gonorrhoeae, Chlamydia trachomatis, Streptococcus viridans*, and group B *Streptococcus*.[31,32] Intra-amniotic infection can clinically manifest itself in very different ways, such as chorioamnionitis or subclinical microbial invasion. The process is a continuum with the signs and symptoms of systemic infection at one end of the spectrum and a completely asymptomatic pregnancy at the other.[33] The findings of a short cervix, preterm labor, and PPROM may occur between those extremes and is believed to be mediated by progressive inflammation. Vaginal infections, such as *Trichomonas vaginalis* and bacterial vaginosis, can contribute to progression through this continuum by at least 2 mechanisms. The first is to instigate the release of cytokines, hydrolytic enzymes, and other proinflammatory agents that increase the local pH and change the vaginal microbiome. The second is to induce local immune modulation that is favorable to other pathologic organisms, such as those listed previously. Both cascading processes have considerable crossover effects and could eventually allow access to the upper genital tract leading to sPTB/PPROM.[34]

Amniocentesis is a means for examining the amniotic fluid for signs of infection through bacterial culture. Other tests routinely used to identify intraamniotic infections include amniotic fluid Gram stain, glucose less than 14 mg/dL, white blood cell count greater than 30/mm^3, and presence of leukocyte esterase.[36] However, an amniocentesis, utilizing these widely available testing criteria will fail to diagnose histologically proven chorioamnionitis in 62% cases. This is likely due to microbial invasion occurring late in the pathophysiologic process.[36] The high sensitivity and low specificity have limited the clinical usefulness of amniocentesis and it should not be required before treatment of a short cervix with cerclage or other therapy.[12,37] However, the diagnosis of chorioamnionitis by standard clinical criteria or amniocentesis is a contraindication to cerclage due to the risk of propagating a potential systemic infection and the associated adverse perinatal outcome.[38] Treatment includes aggressive antimicrobial therapy and usually delivery regardless of gestational age to avoid serious maternal morbidity and mortality. To intervene before the development of systemic infection, assays of proinflammatory agents, such as the cytokine interleukin-6 and the collagen-cleaving enzyme matrix metalloproteinase-8 have been developed as biomarkers for inflammation. Increased levels in the amniotic fluid are consistent with intraamniotic inflammation. However, testing for these biomarkers is limited and not readily available for timely clinical decision making.[39] In the absence of the standard amniotic fluid evidence of chorioamnionitis, patients with a short cervix and evidence of only intraamniotic inflammation are more likely to have a favorable outcome with cerclage therapy.[40] Perhaps the value or amniocentesis lies with the patient who has clinical findings suspicious for chorioamnionitis, but not diagnostic, such as in the case of membrane prolapse into the vagina or cervical dilation at 2 cm or greater.[38] In this circumstance, despite the limited availability of proinflammatory biomarkers, the patient and provider can be reassured with a negative finding on amniocentesis and expect a high rate of success with therapy. In contrast, a positive result consistent with chorioamnionitis would allow for appropriate counseling of patients as to the associated grave prognosis.

Recently, there have been 2 small studies that analyzed the outcomes of patients with amniocentesis-proven intraamniotic infection or inflammation who were treated with long-term (up to 4 weeks) high-dose antibiotics. The first study enrolled 22 second-trimester patients with cervical dilation, and no contractions. About half the patients had amniocentesis evidence of chorioamnionitis and two-thirds received an examination-indicated cerclage. The results included 1 of every 4 delivering extremely premature, 5 total perinatal deaths, and no data on maternal morbidity and mortality.[41] The second study enrolled 62 early third- and late second-trimester patients with preterm labor, about half with evidence of chorioamnionitis by amniocentesis, and 1 of every 6 received a history- or examination-indicated cerclage. Their results showed half delivering extremely premature, limited perinatal mortality data, and no maternal morbidity or mortality data.[42] Both studies reported high rates of resolution of intraamniotic infection and successful prolongation of pregnancy. Because of the wide variety of patients treated, limited data, multiple treatments, small sample size, and limited success, this therapy remains unproven and is not recommended. It should only be contemplated in very select patients with consideration for infectious disease consultation and extensive discussion with respect to the potential adverse outcome for both mother and fetus.

SURGICAL TREATMENT WITH CERCLAGE
McDonald Technique

Cervical cerclage is a surgical procedure in which a suture is placed in the cervix to add support to the cervical stroma. It is typically placed circumferentially around the cervix. There are multiple types of surgical techniques used for suture placement. The McDonald cerclage is the most common technique used in the United States due to ease and efficacy.[43] Regional anesthesia is usually sufficient to allow visualization and placement. The cervical-vaginal junction is identified and the suture is placed as close to the internal cervical os as possible. Because approximately half of the cervical stroma is above the cervical vesical junction the cerclage is typically located in the middle third of the cervix. The actual location can be affected by other factors, including maternal anatomy, obesity, and tissue redundancy.[12,37,44] Lateral suture placement involves identifying the cervical-vaginal fold located in the vaginal fornices, which can be identified by traction and release of the cervix. The suture is placed circumferentially around the cervix. The suture is usually tied directly anterior or posterior and for easier removal (**Fig. 2**). The knot position has not been shown to be a factor in outcome.[45] McDonald cerclage removal is usually done at 36 to 37 weeks. Most cases can be done in an outpatient office and removal allows the potential for vaginal delivery. Occasionally, anesthesia is needed to facilitate adequate exposure. The average time from cerclage removal to delivery is approximately 2 weeks, but a significant portion will deliver within 72 hours.[37,46]

Shirodkar Technique

The Shirodkar procedure is another transvaginal technique commonly used in patients who do not have enough cervical length extending into the vagina for the McDonald technique. This circumstance may be due anatomic variation or due to single or multiple gynecologic procedures of the cervix, such as cone biopsy, loop excision, cryoablation, or other surgical events. Some obstetric care providers prefer this technique as first-line therapy due to the ability to place the circumferential suture closer to the internal os. The Shirodkar technique allows for higher placement by dissecting the bladder and rectum away from the cervix (**Fig. 3**). The vaginal mucosa is incised

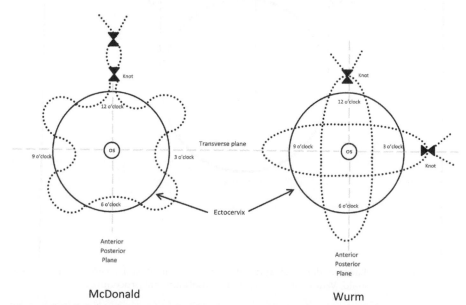

McDonald   Wurm

Fig. 2. Schematic diagram of transvaginal cerclage placement by the McDonald (on the left) and Wurm techniques (on the right).

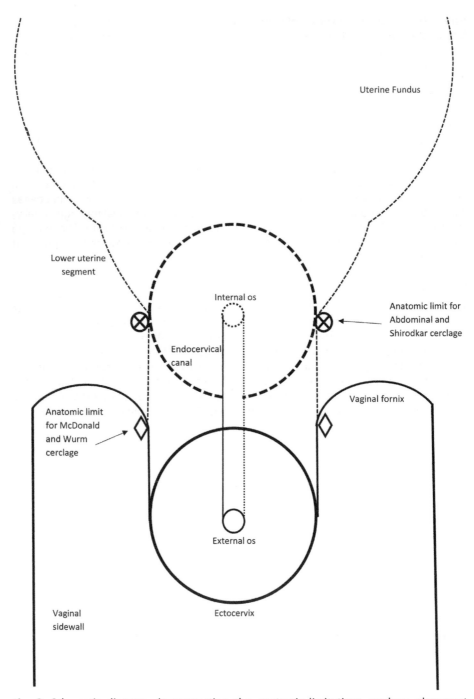

Fig. 3. Schematic diagram demonstrating the anatomic limitations cerclage placement including the McDonald, Wurm, Shirodkar, and transabdominal procedures.

circumferentially at the vesical-cervical junction (approximately the same general area where a McDonald cerclage would be placed) and the bladder is reflected anteriorly. Using the same type of dissection, the rectum is reflected posteriorly and the peritoneum of the rectovaginal pouch displaced superiorly to the level of just above the uterosacral ligaments. Under direct visualization, 2 long Allis type-clamps are placed (one on the right side and the other on the left) with 1 blade in the anterior portion of the dissection and the other blade in the posterior portion. The clamps are closed on the parametrial tissue adjacent to the cervical stroma and medial to the cervical branch of the uterine artery at the level the internal os. When correctly placed, right and left clamps should be at the 9:00 and 3:00 positions, respectively, according to cervical orientation and at the same level as the internal os. The circumferential suture is placed through the cervical tissue on each side just above the tip and medial of each clamp and tied firmly but without tissue strangulation with the knot usually in the 12:00 or 6:00 position. Because of the more extensive dissection associated with the Shirodkar technique, the procedure is potentially more morbid and patient recovery may take longer. The submucosal position of the suture allows it to remain in place, in most circumstances, until completion of childbearing, but can be removed after each pregnancy. Delivery would require caesarean section in the case of desired retention for future pregnancy or by vaginal delivery after removal. Pregnancy loss in the first or early second trimester usually can be treated with dilation and curettage under ultrasound guidance with most Shirodkar sutures allowing passage of an 8 to 10 mm diameter curette. Pregnancy loss in later gestation will require cerclage removal with the potential for extensive dissection or hysterotomy. Like the placement, suture removal will require an additional surgical procedure requiring, at least, regional anesthesia and moderate tissue dissection with increased morbidity compared with the other transvaginal techniques.

There have been several studies that have compared perinatal outcome according to the height of cerclage with respect to cervical length. These studies were done with most patients treated with a McDonald-type of cerclage and the results were mixed.[37,44,47] In addition, the Shirodkar and McDonald techniques have been compared in multiple studies with respect to perinatal outcome, again with mixed results.[12,37,48] Also, different suture types, the number of sutures placed (1 versus 2), knot placement (12:00 versus 6:00; see **Fig. 2**), preoperative studies, including amniocentesis and other testing to rule out infection and/or inflammation, perioperative tocolysis, and antibiotic regimes have also been compared with no significant differences or mixed results. The use of these variations are best administered according to a carefully crafted protocol that allows adjustments to the preference and experience of the health care provider and patient. All these studies would suggest the most important factor to consider would be cerclage placement itself rather than location, method, suture type, knot placement, number of stitches, preoperative testing, perioperative tocolytic, or antibiotic choice.[12,16,37,44,45,47–52]

Wurm Technique

The Wurm procedure is a transvaginal procedure with placement of 2 U-type mattress stitches at the cervical-vaginal reflection. One stitch is placed in the anterior-posterior plane starting at 11:00 through the cervical stroma to 7:00 then looping back from 5:00 to 1:00 and tying at 12:00. The second stitch is placed perpendicular to the first starting at 2:00 to 10:00, looping from 8:00 to 4:00, then tying at 3:00. The suture is usually passed through only the cervical stromal tissue, but in cases where the cervix is thin due to effacement, entering and exiting the endocervical canal often cannot be avoided This technique is not widely used in the United States and is not well studied.

It is mostly used in cases where dilation of the external os is present, such as in the case of examination-indicated cerclage or where a minimal amount of cervical tissue extends into the vagina in lieu of a Shirodkar-type dissection.[53] Removal is similar to the methods for McDonald-type suture (see **Fig. 2**).

Abdominal Cerclage Technique

Abdominal cerclage placement requires peritoneal entry and general anesthesia in most cases. This procedure is associated with the longest recovery time, and has the most potential for maternal morbidity. Most often, this procedure is reserved for transvaginal cerclage failures and significant anatomic defects from congenital disorders or previous obstetric or gynecologic procedures resulting in loss of cervical stromal integrity.[54] Traditionally, abdominal cerclage procedures were completed during pregnancy by open laparotomy through a midline or transverse lower abdominal incision. The timing was usually after 11 weeks when the risk of first trimester loss has passed, when a live fetus with normal aneuploidy screening can be documented, and before the gravid uterus becomes too large (greater than 16 weeks). However, placement in the nonpregnant state and utilization of minimally invasive, including robotic, surgical techniques have become common practice.[55] Regardless of the surgical approach, retroperitoneal dissection of each pelvic sidewall, reflection of the bladder dome anteriorly and inferiorly exposing the lower uterine segment, and identification of the uterine vasculature is required. The suture is placed through the lateral cervical stroma at the level of the internal os at the cervical uterine junction and medial to the cervical branch of the uterine artery similar to the suture position of the Shirodkar procedure (see **Fig. 3**). The knot is tied anteriorly or posteriorly in the midline. The suture is typically left until completion of childbearing. Delivery occurs by caesarean section. Treatment of pregnancy loss is similar to the Shirodkar procedure. Removal requires an additional intraabdominal procedure and general anesthesia. However, minimally invasive techniques or a transvaginal approach with colpotomy, especially with knots tied posteriorly, have been used.

TIMING OF CERCLAGE PROCEDURES

Cerclage procedures can also be classified by the timing of the procedure with many different descriptive terms used in the past. The American College of Obstetrics and Gynecology most recent publication on cervical insufficiency suggested standardized descriptive terms, which are listed below.[11]

HISTORY-INDICATED/PROPHYLACTIC CERCLAGE

History-indicated cerclage describes the procedures usually done in the late first to early second trimester because of previous symptoms. The traditional indications include one or more previous second-trimester losses at 16 weeks or greater. The high success rate should be tempered with the acknowledgment of data suggesting that most patients with a history consistent with cervical insufficiency will not have recurrent preterm birth.[56–59] Although cerclage has been used for sPTB, data supporting its use is limited except with a history of 3 or more sPTB/PPROM.[60] There are other historic risk factors for sPTB/PPROM, including previous cervical surgery, uterine anomalies, and multiple cervical dilation procedures. The positive predictive value of these factors is low and the vast majority of patients with these conditions will deliver at or near term. In addition, singleton patients with these factors have not shown to benefit from history-indicated cerclage in the absence of prior sPTB/PPROM. In addition, cervical surveillance with serial cervical length assessment has not been shown to be of benefit. A single midtrimester cervical length measurement as a part of risk assessment or universal screening is appropriate.[12,61–66] Twins and higher-order multiple gestation also have not shown benefit with history-indicated cerclage.[67,68]

ULTRASOUND-INDICATED CERCLAGE

Ultrasound-indicated cerclage includes those patients who have the ultrasound findings of a cervical length less than 2.5 cm. Some patients have very subtle symptoms such as abdominal cramping, change in vaginal discharge, pelvic pressure, or spotting vaginal bleeding; but most cases are asymptomatic. A short cervix can be found as part of the screening of high-risk patients who have a history of sPTB/PPROM, a universal screening protocol, or incidentally on an ultrasound for other indications. Transvaginal ultrasound is considered the gold standard for cervical length assessment. The guidelines for standardized measurement have been well established.[69] Various other ultrasound parameters have been described, including the width and depth of a funnel (membrane prolapse into the endocervical canal), a U-shape funnel (see **Fig. 1**), presence of dynamic change, and lower uterine segment angle. All are associated with an increased risk of adverse outcome to varying degrees. The cervical length seems to have the strongest inverse relationship to risk of preterm birth and PPROM.[23,70,71]

In singleton pregnancies, a history of previous sPTB/PPROM is the predominant risk factor for sPTB/PPROM. Serial transvaginal cervical length screening from 16 to 24 weeks has been suggested to provide benefit.[14,15] The optimal time between screenings has not been established, but 1- to 4-week intervals have been used with 2-week intervals most commonly used in published reports.[59,72]

Ultrasound-indicated cerclage in patients with a history of sPTB/PPROM less than 34 weeks and a short cervix in the second trimester have demonstrated improved outcome compared with no therapy.[73] However, when compared with history-indicated cerclage, ultrasound-indicted cerclage has similar outcomes. Therefore, patients with less than 3 sPTB/PPROM can be safely followed by serial transvaginal measurements and ultrasound-indicated cerclage as needed. Multiple reports have established the same neonatal results and the maternal benefit of less surgical intervention.[56–59] Several recent studies have shown that patients with a previous cerclage can be safely followed with serial transvaginal cervical length measurements between 16 and 24 weeks with ultrasound-indicated cerclage in cases of a short cervix. The perinatal outcome was comparable with repeat history-indicated cerclage and more than half (57%) delivered at or near term without a cerclage. For singleton pregnancies, these findings would argue against the myth of "once a cerclage, always a cerclage."[58]

Transvaginal cervical length screening may be useful in other situations associated with increased risk of sPTB/PPROM. These include previous cervical surgery, uterine anomalies, history of indicated PTB, late preterm birth (34–36 weeks), and gynecologic procedures associated with forceful cervical dilation. These minor risk factors are associated with a modest increase in probability for sPTB/PPROM and, in the absence of a prior delivery less than 34 weeks, can be safely followed with universal screening or as part of a broader preterm birth prevention program. The development of a short cervix should prompt a standard evaluation to rule out increased uterine activity, placental abruption, and/or intraamniotic infection. In the absence of contraindication, cerclage therapy can be considered similar to patient's with no risk factors described below.

A short cervix in patients without any risk factors (nulliparous or all prior deliveries >37 weeks) will be found incidentally in the second trimester in approximately 2% of patients screened.[74] Ultrasound-indicated cerclage in these patients has shown limited success. However, there may be a subset of patients with an extremely short cervix, defined as less than 1.0 cm, that may benefit from cerclage placement.[73] It should be noted that these patients with an extremely short cervix will have a considerable amount of crossover with the examination-indicated populations. For these reasons, cerclage placement without a history of previous sPTB/PPROM, should be reserved for specific circumstances, including an extremely short cervix and failed or contraindicated medical therapy.[12]

MULTIPLE GESTATION AND ULTRASOUND-INDICATED CERCLAGE

Ultrasound-indicated cerclage in multiple gestation has been an area of considerable controversy, with some studies showing the potential for harm and others showing no evidence of benefit.[12,37,75] However, there have been some studies suggesting benefit in select patients with twins only. This benefit has been limited to those patients with a short cervix, defined as less than 1.5 cm.[76,77] In these circumstances, cerclage placement in twins should be considered. In higher-order multiples, cerclage has not demonstrated benefit regardless of technique or timing.[78]

In patients with a prior multiple gestation complicated by sPTB/PPROM, the risk of recurrent preterm birth in a singleton gestation does not seem to be significantly increased, with an approximately 12% incidence. These findings would suggest that sPTB/PPROM in twins is more a function of multiple gestation. For these reasons, it is appropriate to follow with standard cervical length assessment.[79]

EXAMINATION-INDICATED/RESCUE CERCLAGE

The indications for examination-indicated cerclage (often referred to as rescue cerclage) include visible fetal membranes prolapsed at or near the external os or extending beyond into the vagina on speculum examination with dilation of 1 cm or greater on digital examination regardless of obstetric history. Most studies have shown significant improvement in singleton and twins with cerclage placement usually by the McDonald-type and occasionally abdominal, Shirokar- or Wurm-type procedures.[52,80,81] Care must be taken to minimize membrane manipulation to avoid rupture. Membranes can be reduced by filling the maternal bladder with up to 800 mL of normal saline transurethrally. Transabdominal ultrasound can be used to determine the volume needed to retract the fetal membrane. If a portion of the membrane remains distal to the internal os, then a transcervical 16F Foley catheter with a 30 cc balloon can be placed to elevate the membranes. The bulb is placed just above the internal os and inflated under ultrasound guidance until it reduces the remainder of the membranes and completely obstructs the internal os. Transabdominal amnioreduction procedure under ultrasound guidance has also been used to reduce the membranes. Once the internal os is completely obstructed, the maternal bladder is emptied to facilitate transvaginal cerclage placement. With prolapse of the membranes, preoperative and postoperative Trendelenburg positioning with the maternal feet elevated is often ordered in an effort to reduce pressure on the cervix. The overall benefit of the Trendelenburg position has not yet been determined. Modified activity can be considered, including ambulation as needed to provide for routine personal care, work from home, physical therapy, and mild exercise. Exercise with a short cervix has been shown to be beneficial in some patients and ambulation has shown to be associated with a reduction in pregnancy-related thromboembolic disease.[82] Postoperative cervical surveillance need only consist of single measurement to document positioning of the cerclage and can be timed at 23 to 24 weeks with potential steroid enhancement of fetal lung maturity for findings consistent with cerclage failure. For patients with a cerclage in place, regardless of technique or timing, serial measurements of cervical length have not been shown to be of benefit.[11,12] All patients should be followed by standard high-risk management protocols for sPTB/PPROM prevention, which would include frequent patient contact and education as to the signs and symptoms of preterm labor. Any suspicious finding should investigated in a timely fashion and evaluation could include a speculum and/or digital pelvic examination with or without ultrasound assessment of cervical length as clinically indicated.

CERCLAGE REVISION

On occasion, a cerclage procedure will fail. Although technique and location are often blamed, the cause is most often extrinsic to cervical tissue integrity and may include subclinical uterine activity, chorioamnionitis, and/or placental abruption.[6] Cerclage failure may result in cervical stromal damage, which may be minimal in cases where monofilament suture is used as it usually pulls through the tissue in only 1 or 2 quadrants. When 3- to 5-mm braided tape or multiple sutures are used, the damage can be considerably more extensive. Cerclage revision or reinforcement procedures involve removing the failed suture and placement of second cerclage. Revision procedures have been reported with limited success and are not generally recommended.[83] The exception would be in cases where underlying pathology is ruled out or stabilized and comprehensive informed consent is documented, including the potential for perinatal loss and serious maternal morbidity. These cases should only be done in medical centers with surgeons who are familiar with this type of procedure and preferably use data collection for the purpose of advising patients of their results.

PRETERM PREMATURE RUPTURE OF MEMBRANES WITH A CERCLAGE IN PLACE

On occasion, a patient will experience PPROM with a cerclage in place. If there are signs and/or symptoms of chorioamnionitis, placental abruption, spontaneous labor, or other indication for delivery, the cerclage should be removed with further treatment, including delivery as clinically indicated. In the absence of these signs and symptoms, cerclage removal in PPROM is controversial. Cerclage removal has been associated with earlier delivery and less fetal and maternal infectious morbidity, and cerclage retention has been associated with the opposite. Therefore, treatment should be individualized according to obstetric and infectious history, ease of removal, and maternal autonomy. Some authors have recommended removal after steroid optimization of fetal lung maturity. For patients with an uncertain diagnosis of PPROM or chorioamnionitis, amniocentesis can be considered[12,37,84,85]

MEDICAL THERAPY WITH PROGESTERONE

Medical therapy with progesterone to reduce the risk of sPTB/PPROM can be stratified into 2 broad categories: prevention/prophylaxis and treatment. Prevention begins before the onset of signs or symptoms of sPTB/PPROM, usually at 16 to 20 weeks, and continues to 34 to 37 weeks. Prevention is indicated for patients with a history of sPTB/PPROM before 34 weeks. Prevention with progesterone therapy can also be divided into 2 categories according to route of administration and dosing interval: weekly intramuscular 250 mg or subcutaneous 275 mg injections of 17 alpha-hydroxyprogesterone caproate (17P) or daily 200 mg pharmaceutically compounded suppositories or micronized capsules of intravaginally placed progesterone. Common side effects for progesterone therapy are usually mild and include edema, dizziness, drowsiness, headache, mood changes, and irritation at the site of administration. Contraindications include cardiovascular disease, cerebral vascular accidents, thrombo-embolic disease, breast cancer, reproductive tract cancers, liver disease, and allergic reactions to progestins or the inert components. The mechanism of action for progesterone prevention of sPTB/PPROM is thought to be the inhibitory effect on myometrial cells with respect to limiting prostaglandin synthesis, suppression of oxytocin and prostaglandin receptor formation, and prevention of smooth muscle gap junction formation.[86,87]

WEEKLY INJECTIONS OF 17 ALPHA-HYDROXYPROGESTERONE CAPROATE

Initial studies reported a significant benefit of 17P and it became commercially widely available by 2005.[88] Therapy is usually initiated between 16 and 20 weeks. However, recent studies have called into question the reported benefit of 17P over placebo.[89] Therefore, the use of 17P for PTB/PPROM is not clear at present and should be used only with full disclosure to patients of its potential limitations and availability of alternative therapies.[90] In addition, 17P should not be used for a history of indicated preterm birth at any gestational age. With respect to treatment of short cervix or preterm labor, 17P has not shown benefit and is not recommended.[86,87,91] Weekly injections of 17P are usually discontinued at 36 weeks or earlier.

DAILY VAGINAL PROGESTERONE

Prevention of recurrent sPTB/PPROM with VP has been shown to improve perinatal outcome.[92] A number of studies have shown vaginal progesterone (VP) to be effective in the treatment of patients with a short cervix less than 2.5 cm, including those with of

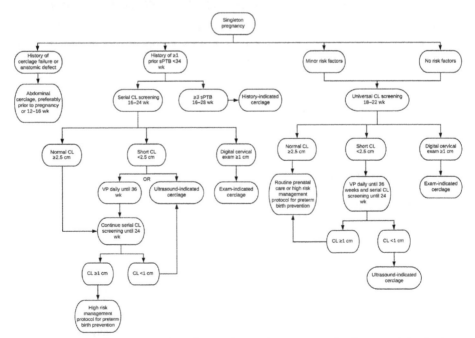

Fig. 4. Flow chart for evidence-based screening and treatment of a short cervix in singleton pregnancies.

history of previous sPTB/PPROM 16 to 33 weeks, minor risk factors, and no risk factors.[93–95] VP has been shown to have similar efficacy compared with cerclage in patients with risk factors and superior in patients with no risk factors.[94,95] For these reasons, VP has been coupled with universal cervical length screening and has been suggested as first-line therapy for the finding of a short cervix.[74] Studies have also shown VP to be most effective when the cervical length is greater than 1 cm.[96] Therefore, singleton universal screening may be helpful in early detection of a short cervix before the onset of symptoms. Cervical surveillance should continue until 24 weeks. If the cervical length decreases to less than 1 cm, then ultrasound-indicated cerclage should be considered.[73] After 24 weeks, for patients with treated VP, further serial ultrasound for cervical length is not required.[11,12] These patients should be followed by standard high-risk management protocols for sPTB/PPROM prevention similar to patients with a cerclage.

The use of VP in twin gestations remains controversial. Recent data suggest a potential for limited benefit in twin gestations. Earlier studies initially questioned benefit. However, as a result of limited efficacy of other treatments, such as 17P, cerclage, and pessary, VP has been considered a potential therapy in twins with a short cervix and a

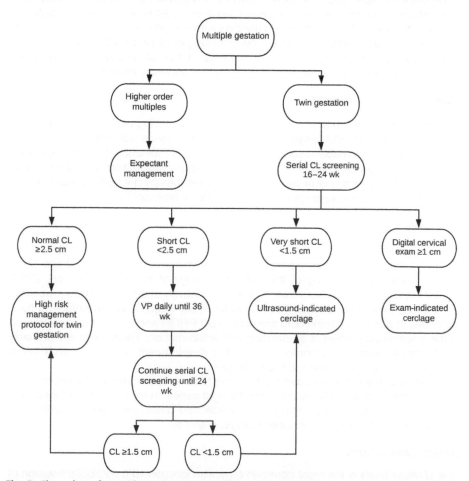

Fig. 5. Flow chart for evidence-based screening and treatment of a short cervix in multiple gestation.

cervical length between 1.5 and 2.5 cm.[97,98] Similar to singletons treated with VP, serial cervical surveillance may provide clinical benefit until 24 weeks. If the cervical length falls below 1.5 cm, then cerclage may be considered.[76,77] After 24 weeks, twins treated with VP can be followed according to management protocols for multiple gestation and without further cervical length screening.

On occasion, a patient receiving preventive therapy with weekly injections of 17P will develop a short cervix and receive daily treatment with VP. Owing to the uncertain benefit of 17P, the rapid increase of bioavailable progesterone levels associated with intravaginal dosing, and the increased potential for progesterone-related side effects, 17P can safely be discontinued in this circumstance.[89] VP is usually discontinued at 36 to 37 weeks.

PESSARY

Vaginal pessaries have long been used in pregnant and nonpregnant populations for treatment of pelvic organ prolapse with a multitude of different designs.[99] The mechanism of action is thought to be its effect on the lower uterine segment angle.[100] Initially, early studies in the United States suggested the benefit of lever-type pessaries placed in select patients with a history of previous sPTB/PPROM.[99] Subsequent larger studies from Europe using a barrel-type pessary showed a promising potential benefit in both singleton and twin pregnancies with a short cervix.[101,102] However, the most recent studies have not shown benefit compared with no therapy.[103,104] For these reasons, pessary placement for patients at risk of recurrent sPTB/PPROM and/or a short cervix in the second trimester is not generally recommended.

COMBINATION TREATMENTS

Various combination therapies have been reported, including cerclage and VP, cerclage and pessary, VP and pessary, and all 3 together. These were all small studies of different types with variable results.[105–108] No doubt, combination therapy used in series or at the same time will be an area of interest to investigators. However, at this time, the lack of vigorous data supporting combined therapy precludes recommendation for their use in the absence of an investigational protocol.[37]

SUMMARY

As we begin to understand the complexities of term and preterm parturition, it becomes clear that the 2 events are separated by much more than gestational age. Great strides in the understanding of the pathophysiology of preterm parturition, sPTB/PPROM, and short cervix have been made in a relatively short time. These processes and intricate interactions remain poorly understood. Regardless, investigators have continued to pursue biomarkers to predict sPTB/PPROM and increase our awareness of the interrelated pathways of infection and inflammation. Treatments are primarily reactionary to anatomic changes, such as the development of a short cervix rather than managing the underlying pathophysiology.

However, in the last 2 decades our treatments have diversified tremendously in an effort to administer the right treatment to the right patient at the right time. Our effort to organize the current understanding for the evidenced-based treatment of a short cervix to prevent sPTB/PPROM is listed in **Figs. 4** and **5**.

CLINICS CARE POINTS

- *U urealyticum* is the most common organism isolated with microbial invasion of the amniotic fluid documented by amniocentesis.

- Interleukin-6 and metalloproteinase-8 are biomarkers diagnostic of intraamniotic inflammation when found at increased levels in the amniotic fluid.
- Assays for placental alpha microglobulin-1 in cervicovaginal secretions have demonstrated efficacy as biomarkers for the prediction of preterm birth in multiple small trials with confirmation by larger multicenter studies pending.
- Patients with less than 3 previous spontaneous preterm births and/or second-trimester losses can be safely followed with serial transvaginal ultrasound cervical length measurements from 16 to 24 weeks and ultrasound-indicated cerclage as needed, rather than history-indicated cerclage, with no difference in perinatal outcome.
- Patients with a history of cerclage placement in a previous pregnancy can also be safely followed with serial cervical length measurements.
- In patients with a singleton pregnancy and a history of previous preterm birth less than 34 weeks, development of a short cervix between 16 and 24 weeks is an indication for surgical treatment with an ultrasound-indicated cerclage or medical treatment with daily vaginal progesterone.
- In patients between 16 and 24 weeks with minor risk factors, no risk factors, or twins and a short cervix (between 1.0–2.4 cm in singletons and 1.5–2.4 cm in twins), daily vaginal progesterone has demonstrated potential benefit.
- In patients between 16 and 24 weeks with a transvaginal cervical measurement of less than 1.0 cm in singletons or 1.5 cm twins, an ultrasound-indicated cerclage should be considered regardless of obstetric history.
- In any patient between 16 and 24 weeks with a cervix dilated to 1–4 cm on digital examination, placement of an examination-indicted cerclage should be considered in both singleton and twin gestations regardless of obstetric history.
- Previous transvaginal cerclage failure or an anatomic defect of the cervix is an indication for abdominal cerclage.
- The evidence to support cerclage placement in high-order multiple gestations (triplets and above) is insufficient.

DISCLOSURE

The authors have nothing to disclose.

REFERENCES

1. Tucker JM, Goldenberg RL, Davis RO, et al. Etiologies of preterm birth in an indigent population: is prevention a logical expectation? Obstet Gynecol 1991; 77(3):343–7.
2. Hamilton BE, Martin JA, Ventura SJ, et al. Births: preliminary data for 2004. Natl Vital Stat Rep 2005;54(8):1–17.
3. Ransom CE, Murtha AP. Progesterone for preterm birth prevention. Obstet Gynecol Clin North Am 2012;39(1):1–16, vii.
4. Cuevas KD, Silver DR, Brooten D, et al. The cost of prematurity: hospital charges at birth and frequency of rehospitalizations and acute care visits over the first year of life: a comparison by gestational age and birth weight. Am J Nurs 2005;105(7):56–64 [quiz: 65].
5. Larma JD, Iams JD. Is sonographic assessment of the cervix necessary and helpful? Clin Obstet Gynecol 2012;55(1):324–35.
6. Rust OA, Atlas RA, Reed J, et al. Revisiting the short cervix detected by transvaginal ultrasound in the second trimester: why cerclage therapy may not help. Am J Obstet Gynecol 2001;185(5):1098–105.

7. Taylor BK. Sonographic assessment of cervical length and the risk of preterm birth. J Obstet Gynecol Neonatal Nurs 2011;40(5):617–31.

8. Iams JD, Johnson FF, Sonek L, et al. Cervical competence as a continuum: a study of ultrasonographic cervical length and obstetric performance. Am J Obstet Gynecol 1995;172(4 Pt 1):1097–103 [discussion: 1104–6].

9. Zemlyn S. The length of the uterine cervix and its significance. J Clin Ultrasound 1981;9(6):267–9.

10. Iams JD, Goldenberg RL, Meis PJ, et al. The length of the cervix and the risk of spontaneous premature delivery. National Institute of Child Health and Human Development Maternal Fetal Medicine Unit Network. N Engl J Med 1996; 334(9):567–72.

11. Cerclage for the management of cervical insufficiency. Practice Bulletin No. 142. American College of Obstetricians and Gynecologists. Obstet Gynecol 2014; 123:372–9.

12. Sperling JD, Dahlke JD, Gonzalez JM. Cerclage use: a review of 3 national guidelines. Obstet Gynecol Surv 2017;72(4):235–41.

13. Andrews WW, Cooper R, Hauth JC, et al. Second-trimester cervical ultrasound: associations with increased risk for recurrent early spontaneous delivery. Obstet Gynecol 2000;95(2):222–6.

14. Sananes N, Meyer N, Gaudineau A, et al. Prediction of spontaneous preterm delivery in the first trimester of pregnancy. Eur J Obstet Gynecol Reprod Biol 2013; 171(1):18–22.

15. Sharvit M, Weiss R, Paz YG, et al. Vaginal examination vs. cervical length—which is superior in predicting preterm birth? J Perinat Med 2017;45(8):977–83.

16. Mackenzie AP, Schatz F, Krikun G, et al. Mechanisms of abruption-induced premature rupture of the fetal membranes: thrombin enhanced decidual matrix metalloproteinase-3 (stromelysin-1) expression. Am J Obstet Gynecol 2004; 191(6):1996.

17. Copper RL, Goldenberg RL, Das A, et al. The preterm prediction study: maternal stress is associated with spontaneous preterm birth at less than thirty-five weeks' gestation. National Institute of Child Health and Human Development Maternal-Fetal Medicine Units Network. Am J Obstet Gynecol 1996; 175(5):1286–92.

18. Gibb W. The role of prostaglandins in human parturition. Ann Med 1998; 30(3):235.

19. Jones SA, Challis JR. Effects of corticotropin-releasing hormone and adrenocorticotropin on prostaglandin output by human placenta and fetal membranes. Gynecol Obstet Invest 1990;29(3):165.

20. Mercer BM, Goldenberg RL, Meis PJ, et al. The preterm prediction study: prediction of preterm premature rupture of the membranes using clinical findings and ancillary testing. Am J Obstet Gynecol 2000;183:738–45.

21. Lee SM, Park KH, Jung EY, et al. Frequency and clinical significance of short cervix in patients with preterm premature rupture of membranes. PLoS One 2017;12(3):e0174657.

22. Goldenberg RL, Mercer BM, Iams JD, et al. The preterm prediction study: patterns of cervicovaginal fetal fibronectin as predictors of spontaneous preterm delivery. National Institute of Child Health and Human Development Maternal-Fetal Medicine Units Network. Am J Obstet Gynecol 1997;177(1):8–12.

23. Esplin MS, Elovitz, Iams JD, et al. Predictive accuracy of serial transvaginal cervical lengths and quantitative vaginal fetal fibronectin levels for spontaneous preterm birth among nulliparous women. JAMA 2017;317(10):1047–56.

24. Keeler SM, Roman AS, Coletta JM, et al. Fetal fibronectin testing in patients with short cervix in the midtrimester: can it identify optimal candidates for ultrasound-indicated cerclage? Am J Obstet Gynecol 2009;200(2):158.e1–6.
25. Kusanovic JP, Espinosz J, Romero R, et al. Clinical significance of the presence of amniotic fluid 'sludge' in asymptomatic patients at high risk for spontaneous preterm delivery. Ultrasound Obstet Gynecol 2007;30(5):706–14.
26. Boyer A, Cameron L, Munoz Maldonado Y, et al. Clinical significance of amniotic fluid sludge in twin pregnancies with a short cervical length. Am J Obstet Gynecol 2014;211(5):506.e1–9.
27. Pirjani R, Moini A, Almasi-Hashiani A, et al. Placental alpha microglobulin-1 (PartoSure) test for the prediction of preterm birth: a systematic review and meta-analysis. J Matern Fetal Neonatal Med 2019;1–13. https://doi.org/10.1080/14767058.2019.1685962.
28. Bahado-Singh RO, et al. Artificial intelligence and amniotic fluid multiomics: prediction of perinatal outcome in asymptomatic women with short cervix. Ultrasound Obstet Gynecol 2019;54(1):110–8.
29. Goldenberg RL, Hauth JC, Andrews WW, et al. Intrauterine infection and preterm delivery. N Engl J Med 2000;342:1500–7.
30. Gomez R, Romero R, Nien JK, et al. A short cervix in women with preterm labor and intact membranes: a risk factor for microbial invasion of the amniotic cavity. Am J Obstet Gynecol 2005;192(3):678–89.
31. Mercer BM, Arheart KL. Antibiotic therapy for preterm premature rupture of the membranes. Semin Perinatol 1996;20(5):426–38.
32. Shim SS, Romero R, Hong JS, et al. Clinical significance of intra-amniotic inflammation in patients with preterm premature rupture of membranes. Am J Obstet Gynecol 2004;191(4):1339–45.
33. Gibbs RS, Romero R, Hiller SL, et al. A review of premature birth and subclinical infection. Am J Obstet Gynecol 1992;166(5):1515–28.
34. Cauci S, Culhane JF. Modulation of vaginal immune response among pregnant women with bacterial vaginosis by *Trichomonas vaginalis*, *Chlamydia trachomatis*, *Neisseria gonorrhoeae*, and yeast. Am J Obstet Gynecol 2007;196(2):133.e1–7.
35. Romero R, Yoon BH, Mazor M, et al. The diagnostic and prognostic value of amniotic fluid white blood cell count, glucose, interleukin-6, and gram stain in patients with preterm labor and intact membranes. Am J Obstet Gynecol 1993;169(4):805–16.
36. Yoon BH, Romero R, Kim CJ, et al. Amniotic fluid interleukin-6: a sensitive test for antenatal diagnosis of acute inflammatory lesions of preterm placenta and prediction of perinatal morbidity. Am J Obstet Gynecol 1995;172(3):960–70.
37. Wood SL, Owen J. Vaginal cerclage: preoperative, intraoperative, and postoperative management. Clin Obstet Gynecol 2016;59(2):270–85.
38. Romero R, Gonzalez R, Sepulveda W, et al. Infection and labor. VIII. Microbial invasion of the amniotic cavity in patients with suspected cervical incompetence: prevalence and clinical significance. Am J Obstet Gynecol 1992;167(4 Pt 1):1086–91.
39. Oh KJ, Park KH, Kim SN, et al. Predictive value of intra-amniotic and serum markers for inflammatory lesions of preterm placenta. Placenta 2011;32(10):732–6.
40. Kiefer DG, Peltier MR, Keeler SM, et al. Efficacy of midtrimester short cervix interventions is conditional on intraamniotic inflammation. Am J Obstet Gynecol 2016;214(2):276.e1–6.

41. Oh KJ, Romero R, Park JY, et al. Evidence that antibiotic administration is effective in the treatment of a subset of patients with intra-amniotic infection/inflammation presenting with cervical insufficiency. Am J Obstet Gynecol 2019; 221(2):140.e1–18.

42. Yoon BH, Romero R, Park JY, et al. Antibiotic administration can eradicate intra-amniotic infection or intra-amniotic inflammation in a subset of patients with preterm labor and intact membranes. Am J Obstet Gynecol 2019;221(2): 142.e1–22.

43. Bartolo S, Garabedian C, Deruelle P, et al. Evaluation of a new technique of prophylactic cervical cerclage simplified from the Shirodkar cerclage: a pilot study. J Gynecol Obstet Hum Reprod 2017;46(4):343–7.

44. Rust OA, Atlas RO, Meyn J, et al. Does cerclage location influence perinatal outcome? Am J Obstet Gynecol 2003;189(6):1688–91.

45. Wood SL, Owen J. Cerclage: Shirodkar, McDonald, and modifications. Clin Obstet Gynecol 2016;59(2):302–10.

46. Bisulli M, Shuhag A, Arvon R, et al. Interval to spontaneous delivery after elective removal of cerclage. Am J Obstet Gynecol 2009;201(2):163.e1–4.

47. Berghella V, Ludmir J, Simonazzi G, et al. Transvaginal cervical cerclage: evidence for perioperative management strategies. Am J Obstet Gynecol 2013; 209(3):181–92.

48. Odibo AO, Berghella V, To M, et al. Shirodkar versus McDonald cerclage for the prevention of preterm birth in women with short cervical length. Am J Perinatol 2007;24(1):55–60.

49. Stafford IA, Kopkin RH, Berra AL, et al. Efficacy of different cerclage suture materials in reducing preterm birth. J Matern Fetal Neonatal Med 2019;1–5. https:// doi.org/10.1080/14767058.2019.1578744.

50. Giraldo-Isaza MA, Fried GP, Hegarty SE, et al. Comparison of 2 stitches vs 1 stitch for transvaginal cervical cerclage for preterm birth prevention. Am J Obstet Gynecol 2013;208(3):209.e1–9.

51. Berghella V, Prasertcharoensuk W, Cotter A, et al. Does indomethacin prevent preterm birth in women with cervical dilatation in the second trimester? Am J Perinatol 2009;26(1):13–9.

52. Atia H, Ellaithy M, Altraigey A, et al. Knot positioning during McDonald cervical cerclage, does it make a difference? A cohort study. J Matern Fetal Neonatal Med 2019;32(22):3757–63.

53. Hefner JD, Patow WE, Ludwig J M. A new surgical procedure for the correction of the incompetent cervix during pregnancy. The Wurm procedure. Obstet Gynecol 1961;18:616–20.

54. Shennan A, Chandiramani M, Bennett P, et al. MAVRIC: a multicenter randomized controlled trial of transabdominal vs transvaginal cervical cerclage. Am J Obstet Gynecol 2020;222(3):261.e1–9.

55. Mourad J, Burke YZ. Needleless robotic-assisted abdominal cerclage in pregnant and nonpregnant patients. J Minim Invasive Gynecol 2016;23(3):298–9.

56. Suhag A, Reina J, Sanapo L, et al. Prior ultrasound-indicated cerclage: comparison of cervical length screening or history-indicated cerclage in the next pregnancy. Obstet Gynecol 2015;126(5):962–8.

57. Abenhaim HA, Tulandi T. Cervical insufficiency: re-evaluating the prophylactic cervical cerclage. J Matern Fetal Neonatal Med 2009;22(6):510–6.

58. Vousden N, Hezelgrave N, Carter J, et al. Prior ultrasound-indicated cerclage: how should we manage the next pregnancy? Eur J Obstet Gynecol Reprod Biol 2015;188:129–32.

59. Brown JA, Pearson AW, Veillon EW, et al. History- or ultrasound-based cerclage placement and adverse perinatal outcomes. J Reprod Med 2011;56(9–10): 385–92.
60. Final report of the Medical Research Council/Royal College of Obstetricians and Gynaecologists multicentre randomised trial of cervical cerclage. MRC/RCOG Working Party on Cervical Cerclage. Br J Obstet Gynaecol 1993;100(6):516–23.
61. Ville Y, Rozenberg P. Predictors of preterm birth. Best Pract Res Clin Obstet Gynaecol 2018;52:23–32.
62. Fischer RL, Sveinbjornsson G, Hansen C. Cervical sonography in pregnant women with a prior cone biopsy or loop electrosurgical excision procedure. Ultrasound Obstet Gynecol 2010;36(5):613–7.
63. Drakeley AJ, Quenby S, Farquharson RG. Mid-trimester loss—appraisal of a screening protocol. Hum Reprod 1998;13(7):1975–80.
64. Granese R, Mantegna S, Mondello S, et al. Preterm birth: incidence, risk factors and second trimester cervical length in a single center population. A two-year retrospective study. Eur Rev Med Pharmacol Sci 2017;21(19):4270–7.
65. Miller ES, Tita AT, Grobman WA. Second-trimester cervical length screening among asymptomatic women: an evaluation of risk-based strategies. Obstet Gynecol 2015;126(1):61–6.
66. Visintine J, Berghella V, Henning D, et al. Cervical length for prediction of preterm birth in women with multiple prior induced abortions. Ultrasound Obstet Gynecol 2008;31(2):198–200.
67. Rafael TJ, Berghella V, Alfirevic Z. Cervical stitch (cerclage) for preventing preterm birth in multiple pregnancy. Cochrane Database Syst Rev 2014;(9):CD009166.
68. Strauss A, Heer IM, Janssen U, et al. Routine cervical cerclage in higher order multiple gestation—does it prolong the pregnancy? Twin Res 2002;5(2):67–70.
69. Boelig RC, Feltovich H, Spitz JL, et al. Assessment of transvaginal ultrasound cervical length image quality. Obstet Gynecol 2017;129(3):536–41.
70. Mella MT, Berghella V. Prediction of preterm birth: cervical sonography. Semin Perinatol 2009;33(5):317–24.
71. Rust OA, Atlas RO, Kimmel S, et al. Does the presence of a funnel increase the risk of adverse perinatal outcome in a patient with a short cervix? Am J Obstet Gynecol 2005;192(4):1060–6.
72. Berghella V, Rafael TJ, Szychowski JM, et al. Cerclage for short cervix on ultrasonography in women with singleton gestations and previous preterm birth: a meta-analysis. Obstet Gynecol 2011;117(3):663–71.
73. Berghella V, Ciardulli A, Rust OA, et al. Cerclage for sonographic short cervix in singleton gestations without prior spontaneous preterm birth: systematic review and meta-analysis of randomized controlled trials using individual patient-level data. Ultrasound Obstet Gynecol 2017;50(5):569–77.
74. Temming LA, Durst JK, Tuuli MG, et al. Universal cervical length screening: implementation and outcomes. Am J Obstet Gynecol 2016;214(4):523.e1–8.
75. Berghella V, Odibo AO, To MS, et al. Cerclage for short cervix on ultrasonography: meta-analysis of trials using individual patient-level data. Obstet Gynecol 2005;106(1):181–9.
76. Roman A, Rochelson B, Fox NS, et al. Efficacy of ultrasound-indicated cerclage in twin pregnancies. Am J Obstet Gynecol 2015;212(6):788.e1–6.
77. Qureshey EJ, Quinones JN, Rochon M, et al. Comparison of management options for twin pregnancies with cervical shortening. J Matern Fetal Neonatal Med 2019;1–7. https://doi.org/10.1080/14767058.2019.1706477.

78. Moragianni VA, Cohen JD, Smith SJ, et al. The role of ultrasound-indicated cerclage in triplets. Ultrasound Obstet Gynecol 2009;34(1):43–6.

79. Menzies R, Li ALK, Murphy KE, et al. Risk of singleton preterm birth after prior twin preterm birth: a cohort study. J Matern Fetal Neonatal Med 2019;1–6. https://doi.org/10.1080/14767058.2019.1581166.

80. Hole J, Tressler T, Martinez F. Elective and emergency transabdominal cervicoisthmic cerclage for cervical incompetence. J Reprod Med 2003;48(8): 596–600.

81. Basbug A, Bayrak M, Dogan O, et al. McDonald versus modified Shirodkar rescue cerclage in women with prolapsed fetal membranes. J Matern Fetal Neonatal Med 2020;33(7):1075–9.

82. Saccone G, Berghella V, Venturella R, et al. Effects of exercise during pregnancy in women with short cervix: secondary analysis from the Italian Pessary Trial in singletons. Eur J Obstet Gynecol Reprod Biol 2018;229:132–6.

83. Contag SA, Woo J, Schwartz, et al. Reinforcing cerclage for a short cervix at follow-up after the primary cerclage procedure. J Matern Fetal Neonatal Med 2016;29(15):2423–7.

84. Aguin E, Van de Ven C, Cordoba M, et al. Cerclage retention versus removal following preterm premature rupture of membranes and association with amniotic fluid markers. Int J Gynaecol Obstet 2014;125(1):37–40.

85. Giraldo-Isaza MA, Berghella V. Cervical cerclage and preterm PROM. Clin Obstet Gynecol 2011;54(2):313–20.

86. Vidaeff AC, Belfort MA. Critical appraisal of the efficacy, safety, and patient acceptability of hydroxyprogesterone caproate injection to reduce the risk of preterm birth. Patient Prefer Adherence 2013;7:683–91.

87. O'Brien JM, Lewis DF. Prevention of preterm birth with vaginal progesterone or 17-alpha-hydroxyprogesterone caproate: a critical examination of efficacy and safety. Am J Obstet Gynecol 2016;214(1):45–56.

88. Meis PJ, Klebanoff M, Thom E, et al. Prevention of recurrent preterm delivery by 17 alpha-hydroxyprogesterone caproate. N Engl J Med 2003;384(13):2379–85.

89. Blackwell SC, Gyamfi-Bannerman C, Biggio JR Jr, et al. 17-OHPC to prevent recurrent preterm birth in singleton gestations (PROLONG study): a multicenter, international, randomized double-blind trial [published ahead of print]. Am J Perinatol 2019. https://doi.org/10.1055/,3400227.

90. Society of Maternal-Fetal Medicine Statement. Use of 17-alpha hydroxyprogesterone caproate for prevention of recurrent preterm birth Society for Maternal-Fetal Medicine. SMFM) Publications Committee; 2019.

91. Keeler SM, Kiefer D, Rochon M, et al. A randomized trial of cerclage vs. 17 alpha-hydroxyprogesterone caproate for treatment of short cervix. J Perinat Med 2009;37(5):473–9.

92. da Fonseca EB, Bitar RE, Carvalho MHB, et al. Prophylactic administration of progesterone by vaginal suppository to reduce the incidence of spontaneous preterm birth in women at increased risk: a randomized placebo-controlled double-blind study. Am J Obstet Gynecol 2003;188(2):419–24.

93. Hassan SS, Romero R, Vidyadhari D, et al. Vaginal progesterone reduces the rate of preterm birth in women with a sonographic short cervix: a multicenter, randomized, double-blind, placebo-controlled trial. Ultrasound Obstet Gynecol 2011;38(1):18–31.

94. Conde-Agudelo A, Romero R, da Fonseca EB, et al. Vaginal progesterone is as effective as cervical cerclage to prevent preterm birth in women with a singleton

gestation, previous spontaneous preterm birth, and a short cervix: updated indirect comparison meta-analysis. Am J Obstet Gynecol 2018;219(1):10–25.
95. Jarde A, Lutsiv O, Beyene J, et al. Vaginal progesterone, oral progesterone, 17-OHPC, cerclage, and pessary for preventing preterm birth in at-risk singleton pregnancies: an updated systematic review and network meta-analysis. BJOG 2019;126(5):556–67.
96. Daskalakis G, Pergialiotis V. A stepwise approach for the management of short cervix: time to evolve beyond progesterone treatment in the presence of progressive cervical shortening. Am J Obstet Gynecol 2019;220(4):404–5.
97. Jarde A, Lutsiv O, Park CK, et al. Preterm birth prevention in twin pregnancies with progesterone, pessary, or cerclage: a systematic review and meta-analysis. BJOG 2017;124(8):1163–73.
98. Rode L, Klein K, Nicolaides KH, et al. Prevention of preterm delivery in twin gestations (PREDICT): a multicenter, randomized, placebo-controlled trial on the effect of vaginal micronized progesterone. Ultrasound Obstet Gynecol 2011; 38(3):272–80.
99. Dharan VB, Ludmir J. Alternative treatment for a short cervix: the cervical pessary. Semin Perinatol 2009;33(5):338–42.
100. Mendoza M, Maiz N, Garcia-Ruiz I, et al. Prediction of preterm birth and adverse perinatal outcomes after cervical pessary placement in singleton pregnancies with short cervical length. J Matern Fetal Neonatal Med 2019;1–7. https://doi.org/10.1080/14767058.2019.1678137.
101. Goya M, de la Calle M, Pratcorona L, et al. Cervical pessary in pregnant women with a short cervix (PECEP): an open-label randomised controlled trial. Lancet 2012;379(9828):1800–6.
102. Goya M, de la Calle M, Pratcorona L, et al. Cervical pessary to prevent preterm birth in women with twin gestation and sonographic short cervix: a multicenter randomized controlled trial (PECEP-Twins). Am J Obstet Gynecol 2016;214(2): 145–52.
103. Dugoff L, Berghella V, Sehdev H, et al. Prevention of preterm birth with pessary in singletons (PoPPS): randomized controlled trial. Ultrasound Obstet Gynecol 2018;51(5):573–9.
104. Berghella V, Dugoff L, Ludmir J. Prevention of preterm birth with pessary in twins (PoPPT): a randomized controlled trial. Ultrasound Obstet Gynecol 2017;49(5): 567–72.
105. Ali MK, Ahmed SE, Sayed GH, et al. Effect of adjunctive vaginal progesterone after McDonald cerclage on the rate of second-trimester abortion in singleton pregnancy: a randomized controlled trial. Int J Gynaecol Obstet 2020;149(3): 370–6.
106. Wolnicki BG, von Wedel F, Mouzakiti N, et al. Combined treatment of McDonald cerclage and Arabin-pessary: a chance in the prevention of spontaneous preterm birth? J Matern Fetal Neonatal Med 2019;33(19):3249–57.
107. Pacagnella RC, Mol BW, Borovac A, et al. A randomized controlled trial on the use of pessary plus progesterone to prevent preterm birth in women with short cervical length (P5 trial). BMC Pregnancy Childbirth 2019;19(1):442.
108. Shor S, Zimerman A, Maymon R, et al. Combined therapy with vaginal progesterone, Arabin cervical pessary and cervical cerclage to prevent preterm delivery in high-risk women. J Matern Fetal Neonatal Med 2019;2:1–5.

INTERVENTIONS

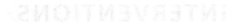

Tocolytic Therapy in Preterm Premature Rupture of Membranes

Hector Mendez-Figueroa, MD*, Suneet P. Chauhan, MD, Hon DSc

KEYWORDS

• Tocolysis • Tocolysis for PPROM • Preterm • Rupture • Membranes

KEY POINTS

- Preterm premature rupture of membranes (PPROM) is defined as the disruption of fetal membranes before the onset of labor and occurring before 37 weeks of gestation.
- A major pitfall to expectant management among cases of PPROM is the possibility of developing significant perinatal complications, such as an intrauterine infection, placental abruption, or even an intrauterine fetal demise.
- Tocolytic therapy thus becomes an interesting alternative, attempting to both decrease uterine contractions and activity that might lead to significant prolongation of pregnancy.
- Reflective of incongruities in the national guidelines, tocolytics are commonly used for women with PPROM. Tocolysis among patients with PPROM remains a poorly studied subgroup among the published literature.
- We will attempt to make some evidence-based conclusions and recommendations based on the available studies and trials.

INTRODUCTION

Preterm premature rupture of membranes (PPROM) is defined as the disruption of fetal membranes before the onset of labor and occurring before 37 weeks of gestation.[1] This complication may be present in approximately 1% to 5% of all pregnancies.[2,3] A well-recognized risk factor for preterm birth, 50% to 75% of women with PPROM deliver within 1 week of membrane rupture.[4] To decrease the sequelae of preterm birth, various management algorithms and protocols are promulgated by national professional societies.[1,5,6]

Prolongation of pregnancies complicated by PPROM is alluring because of the potential of increased benefit to the unborn fetus. It has been well described that

Department of Obstetrics, Gynecology and Reproductive Sciences, McGovern Medical School at The University of Texas Health Science Center at Houston (UTHealth), 6431 Fannin Street, MSB 3.264, Houston, TX 77030, USA
* Corresponding author.
E-mail address: hector.mendezfigueroa@uth.tmc.edu

Obstet Gynecol Clin N Am 47 (2020) 569–586
https://doi.org/10.1016/j.ogc.2020.08.003
0889-8545/20/© 2020 Elsevier Inc. All rights reserved.

obgyn.theclinics.com

gestational age at membrane rupture is inversely related to the latency interval from rupture to delivery.[7,8] Conservative management with a combination of prophylactic antibiotics and corticosteroid therapy improves neonatal outcomes.[9]

A major pitfall to expectant management among cases of PPROM is the possibility of developing significant perinatal complications such as an intrauterine infection, placental abruption, or even an intrauterine fetal demise. Clinically evident infection, a factor known to be detrimental to maternal-fetal dyad, is reported in up to 15% to 25% of women with PPROM.[10,11] Placental abruption, another major complication that could impact maternal-fetal well-being, is reported in 2% to 5% of all PPROM cases.[12,13]

Tocolytic therapy thus becomes an interesting alternative, attempting to both decrease uterine contractions and activity that might lead to significant prolongation of pregnancy. The decision on which medication to use, the preferred route, the dosing, and the length of time for its use are all factors that affect both the acceptability and the effectiveness of the tocolytic. The risk-benefit ratio of such a therapy should clearly favor its use, even when the known side effects are considered.

Tocolytic therapy, used in an acute setting, has been shown to postpone delivery by 24 to 48 hours in cases of preterm birth with intact fetal membranes.[14,15] For example, calcium channel blockers, specifically nifedipine, compared with no treatment or with placebo, have shown a nearly 70% reduction in the rate of birth less than 48 hours following entry to the trial (relative risk [RR] 0.30, with a 95% confidence interval [CI] 0.21–0.43).[14] Betamimetics administered within 48 hours of enrollment also showed a decrease in the risk number of patients delivering within 48 hours close to 40% (RR 0.68, 95% CI 0.53–0.88).[15] Prolongation of pregnancy for 48 hours allows for the administration of medications acknowledged to improve the outcomes among newborns, such as corticosteroids, antibiotics, and magnesium sulfate, specifically for the prevention of cerebral palsy.[16–18] The meta-analyses, which confirmed the benefits of other interventions, reported that utilization of tocolysis neither decreases the rate of preterm birth nor improves the neonatal morbidity and mortality.[14,15] Using betamimetics, for example, failed to achieve a decrease in the rate of preterm birth (RR 0.95; 95% CI 0.88–1.03) or a decrease in the rate of perinatal death (RR 0.84; 95% CI 0.46–1.55) or neonatal death (RR 0.90; 95% CI 0.27–3.00).[15]

When the focus shifts from acute tocolysis to maintenance tocolysis, most publications agree tocolytic therapy beyond 48 hours or repeat course fails to prevent preterm birth and does not improve maternal or neonatal outcomes.[19,20] Maintenance tocolytic therapy with calcium channel blockers revealed no differences in the incidence of preterm birth (risk ratio 0.97; 95% CI 0.87–1.09) or on the rate of neonatal mortality (risk ratio 0.75; 95% CI 0.05–11.76).[19] If there is any rationale for the use of tocolytics among women in preterm birth with intact membranes, the indications appear limited with only partial benefits obtained.

Tocolysis among patients with PPROM remains a poorly studied subgroup among the published literature. It is also important to note that even in modern day obstetrics, there is still much controversy among providers, which leads to a significant variation with the use of these agents among patients with PPROM. A review of several national guidelines by Tsakiridis and colleagues[21] revealed relevant inconsistencies among professional societies regarding the recommendation for the use of tocolytics.

Reflective of incongruities in the national guidelines, tocolytics are commonly used for women with PPROM. In a Web-based survey conducted among maternal-fetal medicine subspecialists, 73% of the 503 respondents stated that tocolysis was their clinical practice when expectantly managing PPROM. The overwhelming majority stated that magnesium sulfate was their main agent and that they generally used the treatment for 48 hours or fewer to obtain the benefit of corticosteroid administration.[22] Similarly, Fellows of the Royal Australian and New Zealand College of Obstetricians and Gynecologists responding to a mailed survey reported that 75% used tocolytics as part of their expectant management protocol for PPROM.[23] In this review, we evaluate and analyze the literature pertaining to the use of these drugs in the expectant management of preterm premature rupture of membranes. We attempt to make some evidence-based conclusions and recommendations based on the available studies and trials.

RELEVANT STUDIES AND TRIALS

The literature addressing the use of tocolytic therapy among patients with PPROM is constrained. In addition, the various tocolytic drugs that have been evaluated and are reported make drawing any conclusions much more challenging. Several other aspects of obstetric care, such as the use of corticosteroids or the administration of antibiotics, differ from one report to the other. Divergent inclusion criteria and different diagnostic standards for identifying a patient with premature rupture of membranes lead to marked heterogeneity among the published studies. Because of these limitations, we present the relevant studies within each subcategory in chronologic order. A summary of the most important trials reported in the literature are summarized in **Table 1**. We first discuss the relevant retrospective studies.

Important Retrospective Analyses

The use of magnesium sulfate for tocolysis in PPROM was evaluated in a retrospective analysis by Fortunato and colleagues.[24] Fifty women were treated with a management protocol comprising intravenous magnesium sulfate used as therapeutic tocolysis and oral terbutaline used as prophylactic tocolysis in combination with prophylactic antibiotic administration. Compared with the 57 women in the control arm, this management protocol led to a significantly longer latency phase, 7.34 days versus 1.86 days, $P<.01$. The rate of postpartum infection was similar, and the rate of neonatal infectious morbidity was also comparable between the groups.

Magnesium sulfate administration for tocolysis was once again evaluated retrospectively by Jazayeri and collaborators.[25] The investigators included patients with PPROM less than 34 weeks of gestation who had received corticosteroids and antibiotics for 7 days. Thirty-six patients received magnesium sulfate tocolysis and were matched to patients with PPROM at a similar gestational age. This analysis revealed that latency was longer in patients who did not receive tocolysis, 60 hours versus 127 hours, $P<.01$. Patients not receiving tocolytics remained pregnant at 48 hours (53% vs 78%, $P = .03$) and at 7 days (8% vs 44%, $P<.01$) at a higher rate. Rates of chorioamnionitis and other adverse neonatal outcomes were similar between the groups.

In 2004, Combs and colleagues[26] reported their results of a retrospective analysis testing aggressive tocolysis after PPROM. They included patients with PPROM before 34 weeks and used a historical cohort as the control group. All patients received corticosteroids for fetal lung maturity and prophylactic ampicillin intravenously. Several agents and dosing of tocolytics were used to suppress uterine activity. Aggressive tocolysis after PPROM led to complications or side effects in almost 20% of all patients. Aggressive therapy was unsuccessful in increasing latency (3.8 days vs 4.5 days, $P = .16$), gestational age at delivery (30.1 vs 30.7 weeks, $P = .55$) or in decreasing neonatal morbidity or death.

Kulmala and Phupong[27] reported a retrospective analysis of 61 women treated with terbutaline compared with 102 women in the control group. Women with a singleton

Table 1
Relevant studies on tocolytics among patients with PPROM

Author/Year Published	Sample Size	Case Group (Tocolytics)	Control Group	Design	Cohorts	Primary Outcome	Principal Finding
Christensen et al,[31] 1980	30	14 IV ritodrine	16	RCT	• Singleton pregnancies • 28–36 wk gestation • Dilated <4 cm	Length of latency period	• More women delivered within 24 h in placebo group (P<.05) • Length of pregnancy after 24 h was the same • No difference in neonatal outcomes
Levy and Warsof,[32] 1985	42	21 Oral ritodrine	21	RCT	• Singleton pregnancies • 25–34 wk gestation	Length of latency period	• Mean latent period of approximately 10 d longer when Ritodrine was used • Pregnant 1 wk - 47.6% ritodrine vs 14.2% no treatment
Dunlop et al,[36] 1986	48	24 Oral ritodrine	24	RCT	• Singleton gestations • 26–34 wk • No uterine contractions	Mode of delivery, neonatal outcomes	• No difference in both primary outcomes
Garite et al,[33] 1987	79	39 Oral ritodrine	40	RCT	• Singleton pregnancies • 25–30 6/7 wk	Length of latency period	• No difference in the interval to delivery, reaching 32 wk, rate maternal morbidity or GA at delivery
Weiner et al,[34] 1988	75	33 Betamimetics and Magnesium sulfate	42	RCT	• Singleton pregnancies • <34 wk	Length of latency period	• GA at delivery, CS rate, maternal infection rates and interval from membrane rupture were all similar • No difference in neonatal outcomes

Study							Results
Fortunato et al,[24] 1990	112	57	Retrospective	55 IV mag for therapeutic PO terbutaline for prophylaxis	• Singleton pregnancies • <37 wk	Length of latency period	• 44% tocolytic vs 10% control undelivered at 5 d, latency was 7.3 vs 1.9 d (P<.01) • No improvement in maternal or infant outcomes
Matsuda et al,[35] 1993	81	42	RCT	39 ritodrine with or without magnesium sulfate	• Singleton pregnancies • 23–35 wk	Length of latency period	• Delivery was significantly delayed for 48 h, 7 d and beyond 35 wk with treatment • The incidence of a low Apgar score, need for artificial ventilation, and infectious morbidity was higher in the treated group
Decavalas et al,[37] 1994	241	105	RCT	136 IV beta-mimetic	• 26 and 35 wk	Length of latency period	• No differences in the latency period • Risk of chorioamnionitis (RR 2.47, 95% CI 1.42–4.66) and endometritis (RR 1.74, 95% CI 1.10–2.75) higher with treatment
How et al,[38] 1998	145	67	RCT	78 IV magnesium sulfate	• Singleton and twins • 24 and 34 completed weeks	Improvement in neonatal outcomes	• No significant differences in GA at delivery, latency, rate of chorioamnionitis, birthweight, days in NICU, neonatal sepsis or neonatal mortality

(continued on next page)

Table 1
(continued)

Author/Year Published	Sample Size	Case Group (Tocolytics)	Control Group	Design	Cohorts	Primary Outcome	Principal Finding
Jazayeri et al,[25] 2003	72	36 IV Magnesium sulfate	36	Retrospective	• Singleton pregnancies • <34 wk	Delivery within 48 h	• Patients not on tocolytics had longer latency, more likely to remain pregnant >48 h and more than a week
Combs et al,[26] 2004	122	59 Several tocolytics	63	Retrospective	• Singleton pregnancies • <34 wk	Length of latency period	• Aggressive tocolysis causes significant side effect without any benefit in increased latency or neonatal morbidity
Ehsanipoor et al,[39] 2011	50	27 oral indomethacin	23	RCT	• Singleton pregnancies • 24–31 6/7 wk	Delivery within 48 h	• There were no differences in the proportion of subjects remaining pregnant beyond 48 h
Kulmala et al,[27] 2012	163	61 IV terbutaline then PO	102	Retrospective	• Singleton pregnancies • 28 and 34 wk • Dilation <4 cm	Length of latency period	• Similar median latency period (78 vs 75 h, $P = .44$) • Percentage of patients undelivered at 48 h was higher in the terbutaline group • Infectious newborn morbidity was higher in the terbutaline group (40.9% vs 22.5% $P = .01$)

Study							Findings
Galyean et al,[40] 2014	56	32 cerclage removal	24	RCT	• 22 wk 0 d and 32 wk 6 d • Previous McDonald or Shirodkar cerclage • Singleton and twins	Prolongation of pregnancy by at least 1 wk, rate of chorioamnionitis	• There was no difference in primary outcome (removal 56.3%; retention 45.8%, $P = .59$); or chorioamnionitis (removal 25.0%; retention 41.7%, $P = .25$) • There was no difference in rate of composite neonatal outcomes, fetal/neonatal death or GA at delivery
Horton et al,[28] 2014	1259	621 IV magnesium sulfate	638	Retrospective	• Singleton pregnancy • 24 and 31 6/7 wk • No evidence of labor	Delivery within 48 h, delivery within 7 d	• The rate of delivery < 48 h was not different (22.2% and 20.7%, $P = .51$) • Delivery < 7 d was similar (55.4% and 51.4%, $P = .16$) • Median latency was also similar • Composite neonatal outcomes were similar between groups
Combs et al,[42] 2015	152	74 17-OHP	78	RCT	• Singleton pregnancies • 23 0/7–30 6/7 wk	Reaching a favorable gestational age (34 0/7 wk GA or documentation of FLM 32 0/7–33 6/7 wk)	• The primary outcome was achieved in 3% of the 17-OHP group and 8% of the placebo group ($P = .18$) • There was no significant in randomization-to-delivery interval or composite adverse perinatal outcome

(continued on next page)

Table 1
(continued)

Author/Year Published	Sample Size	Case Group (Tocolytics)	Control Group	Design	Cohorts	Primary Outcome	Principal Finding
Nijman et al,[43] 2016	50	25 oral nifedipine	25	RCT	• Singleton and twin gestations • No contractions • 24 0/7–33 6/7 wk	Composite adverse perinatal outcome (perinatal death, BPD, PVL > grade 1, IVH > grade 2, NEC > stage 1 or culture proven sepsis)	• The adverse perinatal outcome occurred in 9 neonates (33.3%) in the nifedipine group and 9 neonates (32.1%) in the placebo group (RR 1.04, 95% CI 0.49–2.2)
Lorthe et al,[29] 2017	803	596 several tocolytics	207	Retrospective	• Singleton pregnancies • 24–32 wk	Survival to discharge without severe morbidity, latency >48 h, histologic chorioamnionitis	• No difference in neonatal survival without severe morbidity (86.7% vs 83.9%, $P = .39$), latency >48 h (75.1% vs 77.4%, $P = 0 .59$), or histologic chorioamnionitis (50.0% vs 47.6%, $P = .73$)
Jung et al,[30] 2018	184	143 IV magnesium sulfate	41	Retrospective	• Singleton pregnancies • 23–31 6/7 wk	Prolong pregnancy, improvement in maternal outcomes or perinatal outcomes	• The latency period was significantly longer in the MgSO4 group compared with control (7.9 ± 9.0 vs 4.0 ± 6.0 d, $P<.01$) • MgSO4 therapy led to decreased stillbirth and perinatal mortality

Abbreviations: BPD, bronchopulmonary dysplasia; CI, confidence interval; FLM, fetal lung maturity; GA, gestational age; IV, intravenous; IVH, intraventricular hemorrhage; MgSO4, magnesium sulfate; NEC, necrotizing enterocolitis; NICU, neonatal intensive care unit; PO, oral; PPROM, preterm premature rupture of membranes; PVL, periventricular leukomalacia; RCT, randomized controlled trial; RR, relative risk; 17-OHP, 17-hydroxyprogesterone caproate.

pregnancy complicated by PPROM diagnosed between 28 and 34 weeks and dilated to less than 4 cm were included. All patients were administered corticosteroids for fetal lung maturity and received prophylactic antibiotics for 2 days intravenously and 5 days orally. The patients in the treatment arm received terbutaline intravenously for 48 hours after admission and then switched to oral terbutaline until contractions stopped. The median latency period was comparable between the groups (78 hours vs 75 hours, $P = .44$); however, the rate of patients not delivered within 48 hours was significantly higher in the terbutaline group (78% vs 62%, $P = .03$). Noteworthy is that neonatal infectious morbidity was higher among patients in the terbutaline group (40% vs 22% $P = .01$).

In one of the largest retrospective studies reported, Horton and colleagues[28] reported the results of a secondary analysis of the trial evaluating the use of magnesium sulfate to prevent cerebral palsy. In women with a singleton pregnancy diagnosed with PPROM between 24 and 31 6/7 weeks' gestation without evidence of labor, magnesium sulfate was administered intravenously first as a 6-g bolus, followed by an infusion of 2 g per hour for 12 hours. The primary outcomes were delivery within 48 hours and delivery within 7 days from randomization. A total of 621 women received magnesium sulfate and were compared with 638 controls. All patients received antenatal corticosteroids, no other tocolytics were permitted in the parent trial. The rate of delivery before 48 hours (22.2% and 20.7%, $P = .51$) and delivery within 7 days (55.4% and 51.4%, $P = .16$) were not different between the groups. Median latency was also similar (6.0 days vs 6.6 days, $P = .29$), there was no difference in the rate of the composite neonatal outcome.

Lorthe and colleagues[29] reported the results of a secondary analysis of a national, population-based, prospective cohort of preterm infants recruited in France. Included in this analysis were women with a singleton gestation and PPROM at 24 to 32 weeks' gestation. The investigators used a composite neonatal adverse outcome as the primary endpoint. Several tocolytic agents were used in this study, including the oxytocin-receptor blocker, atosiban. Close to 90% of participants received corticosteroids for fetal lung maturity, and more than 95% received antibiotics. The median latency period was similar between the groups (6 vs 5 days, $P = .26$) and the rate of pregnancy prolongation by 48 hours (75.1% vs 77.4%, $P = .59$). More importantly, the rates of neonatal survival without severe morbidity (86.7% vs 83.9%, $P = .39$) and histologic chorioamnionitis (50.0% vs 47.6%, $P = .73$) were also similar.

The results of a retrospective analysis done in Korea were reported in 2018. Investigators evaluated the perinatal outcomes of pregnancies complicated by PPROM from 23 0/7 weeks to 31 6/7 weeks that were treated with intravenous magnesium sulfate for tocolysis.[30] Prophylactic antibiotics and corticosteroids were routinely administered. The latency period was noted to be significantly longer in the magnesium sulfate group (7.9 vs 4.0 days, $P<.01$). Magnesium administration also led to a significant decrease in the rate of both stillbirth (1.4% vs 14.6%, $P<.01$) and perinatal mortality (7% vs 19.5%, $P = .03$).

Prospective Trials that did Not Include the Use of Corticosteroids

Because of the intrinsic bias present in retrospective studies, few evidence-based conclusions may be inferred. Prospective data can give a better assessment of the rate and the incidence of several clinically important complications. Trials evaluating the use of tocolytics and other agents aimed at prolonging pregnancy among patients with PPROM, dichotomized by their inclusion of corticosteroid therapy, are presented chronologically.

In 1980, Christensen and colleagues[31] reported the results on one of the first randomized controlled trials testing the use of tocolytics among patients with PPROM. They recruited 30 patients with singleton pregnancies complicated by PPROM between 28 and 36 weeks' gestation and were found to be less than 4 cm dilated on admission and used intravenous ritodrine for 24 hours followed by an oral course after this initial infusion as their intervention. No antibiotics or corticosteroids for fetal lung maturity were administered for the participants. They reported that none of the 14 participants in the ritodrine group were delivered within 24 hours compared with 6 of the 16 in the placebo group (P<.05). However, after this initial 24-hour period, the length of pregnancy was similar between the groups. The investigators also noted that there was no difference in neonatal outcomes.

In a study conducted in Virginia, 42 women with a singleton pregnancy complicated by PPROM between 25 and 34 weeks' gestation were randomized to the use of oral ritodrine as tocolysis.[32] Twenty-one patients assigned to the intervention received 10 mg of oral ritodrine every 4 hours until the onset of labor. No prophylactic antibiotics or corticosteroids were administered to the groups. Patients receiving the tocolytic agent had a mean latency period close to 10 days, significantly longer than the control group (P = .028). The percentage of patients still pregnant 1 week after randomization was also significantly different: 47.6% in the oral ritodrine group versus 14.2% in the control arm, P = .045. The limited number of maternal and neonatal outcomes evaluated revealed no differences between both study groups.

Evaluating women from 25 to 30 weeks' gestation, Garite and colleagues[33] assessed the use of ritodrine tocolysis during the expectant management of PPROM. Patients assigned to the intervention group received intravenous ritodrine when 3 or more contractions developed in a 20-minute period, the dose was titrated depending on the contraction pattern observed. Once the clinician decided that labor had been halted, the patient was switched to oral ritodrine at a dose of 10 mg every 3 hours. The intravenous infusion could be repeated a second time if necessary, but once 32 weeks was reached, no more tocolytic was administered. No corticosteroids or prophylactic antibiotics were dispensed to either study group. A total of 79 patients were recruited with 39 being assigned to the tocolytic group. The investigators reported no difference in the interval between rupture of membranes and delivery between the 2 groups, the percentage of patients still pregnant after 48 hours was 77% in the treatment group and 75% in the control group, P>.05. There was also no difference in the percentage of patients reaching 32 weeks of gestation. No statistical difference was seen in the rates of maternal morbidity. Birth weights and gestational ages at delivery were similar between the groups.

Women diagnosed with PPROM before 34 weeks gestation with no evidence of infection were enrolled in a randomized controlled trial conducted in Iowa from 1984 to 1986.[34] Patients assigned to the intervention group had tocolysis started once contractions were noted to be greater than 3 in 1 hour and was discontinued if the patient was diagnosed with an intrauterine infection, was found to be more than 4 cm dilated, or developed intolerance to the tocolytic drug because of side effects. Several agents were permitted in the trial, including ritodrine, terbutaline, and magnesium sulfate. The initial drug was a beta-mimetic for most patients and magnesium was reserved for cases in which uterine activity could not be controlled with the initial agent. No corticosteroids were administered for fetal lung maturity, antibiotics were only administered for clinically evident infections. After randomizing 109 patients, 34 were excluded because of protocol violation, not receiving the tocolytic therapy, withdrawing from the study, or were found to have a multiple gestation. A total of 33 women were assigned to the treatment arm, 50% of these women received 2 tocolytic agents. The interval from membrane rupture to delivery, the gestational age at delivery, rate of cesarean delivery, and number of cases diagnosed with a maternal infection were all found to be similar. There was also no difference in all neonatal outcomes evaluated. On a subgroup analysis, the investigators found that when tocolytics were administered before 28 weeks' gestation, this intervention may increase the period of latency in a pregnancy by 5 additional days.

Matsuda and colleagues[35] reported the results of a randomized controlled trial that enrolled 81 women diagnosed with PPROM. Thirty-nine patients assigned to the tocolytic arm of the trial received ritodrine with or without magnesium sulfate and antibiotic therapy. No corticosteroids were administered for fetal lung maturity. The investigators reported that 87% of the patients in the tocolytic group were still pregnant after 48 hours compared with 50% in the control group, $P<.01$. They also noted a statistically significant difference in the number of pregnant women at 7 days, 39% versus 12%. Of note, the rate of low 5-min Apgar scores of less than 7 (18% vs 0%), the need for artificial ventilation (41% vs 17%), and the diagnosis of infectious morbidity (39% vs 17%) in the newborn were more common in the treated group than in the non-treated group.

Prospective Trials that Included the Use of Corticosteroids

Dunlop and colleagues[36] reported the outcomes of a randomized controlled trial, evaluating the use of ritodrine and cephalexin in the expectant management of PPROM. The investigators created 4 groups for comparison: Group 1 received no ritodrine or cephalexin; group 2 received ritodrine and cephalexin; group 3 received ritodrine but no cephalexin and group 4 received cephalexin but no ritodrine. Corticosteroids were administered to all participants. They assigned mode of delivery and neonatal outcomes as their primary endpoint. The investigators found no difference between the groups regarding the components of the primary outcome.

In one of the largest randomized controlled trials reported to date which was conducted over a 7-year period, 241 women diagnosed with PPROM from 26 to 35 weeks' gestation were assigned to receive either a 48-hour course of tocolytics or a more aggressive tocolytic management protocol.[37] Steroids were administered on a weekly basis to all patients enrolled between 27 and 34 weeks. Patients assigned to the 48-hour course of tocolytics would receive intravenous beta-mimetic tocolysis only if contractions developed and was continued until the second dose of corticosteroids was administered. Women in the aggressive tocolytic arm received intravenous beta-mimetic tocolysis from admission and was continued until delivery. The differences in the latency period were not statistically significant between the groups. The risk of infectious morbidity was higher among women assigned to the aggressive tocolysis. Twelve subjects in the 48-hour group (11.4%) and 40 in the aggressive tocolysis group (29.4%) developed chorioamnionitis (RR 2.47, 95% CI 1.42–4.66, $P<.01$). Rates of endometritis has a similar pattern, 19% in the 48-hour group versus 33.3% in the aggressive management arm (RR 1.74, 95% CI 1.10–2.75, $P<.05$).

In another randomized trial published in 1998, patients diagnosed with PPROM from 24 to 34 completed weeks were randomized to receive aggressive tocolytic therapy compared with no tocolytic therapy.[38] For this study, aggressive tocolytic therapy was initiated when 6 or more contractions were noted in 1 hour and consisted of magnesium sulfate administered intravenously using a 6-g loading dose followed by a maintenance dose of 2 g per hour. The dose was titrated depending on the frequency of contractions until 3 contractions or fewer were noted on the monitor. All patients received prophylactic antibiotics consisting of ampicillin, or clindamycin continued until results for vaginal cultures were obtained. Corticosteroids for fetal lung maturity were administered on a weekly basis until delivery or confirmation of fetal lung maturity. Eight twin gestations were included in this trial. No statistically significant difference between the groups was observed regarding latency from rupture to delivery, a median of 3 days versus 4 days. There was also no difference in the rate of chorioamnionitis, birth weight, the number of days admitted to the neonatal intensive care unit, number of days on oxygen or ventilatory support, the frequency of hyaline membrane disease, diagnosis of neonatal sepsis, or neonatal mortality.

Using indomethacin as a tocolytic agent for patients with PPROM was evaluated in a trial conducted from 2000 to 2005.[39] Women were included if they had a singleton pregnancy complicated by PPROM between 24 0/7 weeks and 31 6/7 weeks and has no evidence of labor or infection. All participants received corticosteroids for fetal lung maturity and prophylactic antibiotics which consisted of intravenous ampicillin/sulbactam for 48 hours followed by oral amoxicillin/clavulanate for 5 days. Patients in the treatment arm received indomethacin 50 mg rectally followed by 25 mg orally every 6 hours for 48 hours. The control arm received a placebo following the same treatment schedule. A total of 50 patients were randomized, of these 27 were allocated to the indomethacin arm. The primary outcome of this trial was to assess rates of delivery within 48 hours of starting the study drug. The investigators concluded that there were no differences in the proportion of subjects remaining pregnant beyond 48 hours, 92% in the placebo arm versus 91% in the treatment arm (RR 1.01 95% CI 0.84–1.21). They also reported no difference in the latency period using a Kaplan-Meier survival analysis. Neonatal outcomes were all similar between the groups.

The benefit of cerclage retention among patients with PPROM has remained controversial. Attempting to answer this question, Galyean and colleagues[40] designed a randomized controlled trial to assess cerclage removal versus retention. Women with a cerclage placed before 24 weeks and diagnosed with PPROM between 22 0/7 weeks and 32 6/7 weeks were included. Both twins and singleton gestations were included in the trial. In this trial, expectant management consisted of corticosteroid administration for fetal lung maturity, prophylactic antibiotics consisting of 2 days of intravenous therapy followed by 5 days of oral treatment and administration of magnesium sulfate for the prevention of cerebral palsy. No tocolytics were administered to either arm. The trial was stopped early after a futility analysis was performed. A total of 58 patients were randomized with 24 assigned to the cerclage retention group. There was no statistical significance in primary outcome or prolongation of pregnancy by 1 week, between the groups (56.3% removal vs 45.8% retention, $P = .59$). The rate of chorioamnionitis were also similar (25% removal vs 41.7% retention, $P = .25$). There was no statistical difference in the rates of composite neonatal outcomes, fetal/neonatal death or the gestational age at delivery.

Using 17-hydroxyprogesterone caproate (17-OHP) to prevent preterm birth has become common practice in the United States.[41] Progesterone has been shown to reduce spontaneous uterine activity in in vitro models. The benefit of 17-OHP among patients with PPROM as an agent for pregnancy prolongation was evaluated in a multi-centered, double-blind, placebo-controlled trial conducted between 2011 to 2014.[42] Singleton pregnancies between 23 0/7 weeks and 30 6/7 weeks not previously on any form of progesterone eligible for expectant management were included. Patients were assigned to receive weekly 17-OHP or an identical placebo until 34 weeks. Corticosteroid administration for fetal lung maturity was given and a rescue course was permitted within the trial. Prophylactic antibiotics and magnesium sulfate to prevent cerebral palsy were administered. The decision on the use of tocolytic therapy was left to the discretion of the treating provider. After enrolling 152 patients, the trial was stopped early for futility. The primary outcome, continuation of pregnancy until either 34 0/7 weeks of gestation or documentation of fetal lung maturity at 32 0/7 to 33 6/7 weeks of gestation, was achieved in 3% of the treatment group versus 8% of the placebo group (P = .18). There were no significant differences between the groups regarding the randomization-to-delivery interval (17.1 vs 17.0 days, P = .76) or the rate of composite adverse perinatal outcome (63% vs 61%, P = .93).

The use of calcium channel blockers as a tocolytic agent was assessed in a nationwide multicenter randomized placebo-controlled trial conducted in The Netherlands.[43] Women with PPROM a gestational age between 24 0/7 and 33 6/7 weeks with no signs of active labor were randomized to receive oral nifedipine 20 mg given every 6 hours or placebo administered until active labor developed, the patient reached 34 weeks' gestation or a maximum of 18 days of therapy was achieved. Antenatal corticosteroids, prophylactic antibiotics, and magnesium sulfate for cerebral palsy prevention were administered to both groups. Using a composite neonatal outcome as a primary endpoint, a sample size of 120 patients was calculated. The trial was stopped early due to slow recruitment. The primary outcome occurred in 9 of the 25 children in the nifedipine group (33.3%) versus 9 children of the 25 children in the placebo group (32.1%) (RR 1.04; 95% CI 0.43–2.5). The median gestation age at delivery, latency period from rupture to delivery and rate of pregnancy after 48 hours of study drug initiation were similar between the groups. Kaplan-Meier survival analysis was also not significant.

META-ANALYSES

At least 3 meta-analyses have attempted to summarize the data regarding the use of tocolytics or other agents for pregnancy prolongation among patients with PPROM. Because most randomized controlled trials assessing tocolytics in PPROM failed to administer agents known to improve perinatal outcomes such as corticosteroids, their conclusions are severely limited and may not apply to modern obstetrics. Also, significant heterogeneity and reporting bias is noted among the trials evaluated for these publications (**Table 2**).

One of the first attempts to consolidate the literature and reach evidence-based conclusions was conducted by Ohlsson in 1989.[44] The investigator evaluated all published randomized controlled trials and assessed several aspects of the treatment of PPROM, including the use of tocolytics. Regarding tocolysis alone, the investigator identified a total of 4 trials. After merging all participants, the review revealed that tocolytic therapy did not have any proven benefit to the mother or the newborn and therefore should not be used outside the setting of a randomized controlled trial.

A more recent review was conducted in 2014 by Mackeen and colleagues.[45] The investigators included all pregnant women with a singleton pregnancy, diagnosed with PPROM between 23 weeks to 36 weeks and 6 days and treated with any tocolytic therapy that was eventually compared with either no tocolytic, placebo, or another other tocolytic agent. They identified a total of 8 trials in the literature that enrolled 408 women. When tocolysis was compared with no therapy (7 trials, n = 402 women), the intervention was associated with a longer latency period (mean difference of 73 hours; 95% CI 20.21–126.03) and fewer births within 48 hours of inclusion (RR 0.55; 95% CI 0.32–0.95). However, the use of tocolysis was not associated with an improvement in the rate of perinatal mortality (9.7% vs 5.8%; RR 1.67; 95% CI 0.85–3.29) and was actually associated with an increase in the rate of 5-minute Apgar score less than 7 (RR 6.05; 95% CI 1.65–22.23) and with an increased need for mechanical ventilation of the newborn (RR 2.46; 95% CI 1.14–5.34).

Table 2
Relevant meta-analyses on agents designed for pregnancy prolongation among patients with PPROM

Author/Year Published	# Trials Included	Total Population	Cohorts	Primary Outcome	Principal Finding
Ohlsson,[44] 1989	4	199	• Singleton pregnancies • 25–36 wk gestation	To evaluate the effect of several interventions used for PPROM	• Tocolysis is not effective in prolonging pregnancy beyond 24 h • Tocolytics cannot be recommended due to their lack of benefit
Mackeen et al,[45] 2014	8	408	• Singleton pregnancies • 23–36 6/7 wk gestation	Perinatal mortality	• Tocolysis was not associated with a significant effect on perinatal mortality (RR 1.67; 95% CI 0.85–3.29). • Tocolysis was associated with longer latency (mean difference 73.12 h; 95% CI 20.21–126.03) • Tocolysis was associated with increased 5-min Apgar < than 7 (RR 6.05; 95% CI 1.65–22.23) • Tocolysis in PPROM < 34 wk was associated with a significant increase in the risk of chorioamnionitis
Quist Nelson et al,[46] 2018	6	545	• Singleton pregnancies • GA < 37 wk	Time from randomization until delivery	• Progesterone administration was not associated with prolonging latency period (mean difference 0.11 d, 95% CI −3.30–3.53) • There was no difference in maternal or neonatal outcomes

Abbreviations: CI, confidence interval; GA, gestational age; PPROM, preterm premature rupture of membranes; RR, relative risk.

The use of progesterone as an agent for pregnancy prolongation among patients with PPROM has been evaluated in a meta-analysis that included 6 trials (n = 545 patients).[46] The investigators included all studies that had singleton pregnancies with the diagnosis of PPROM before 37 weeks that evaluated the use any type of progesterone administered via any route. The primary outcome for this analysis was the time from randomization to delivery. Four of the included trials were conducted in the United States. Four trials evaluated 17 - hydroxyprogesterone caproate only. Corticosteroids for fetal lung maturity were used in all 6 trials. The investigators concluded that there was no difference in the length of latency (mean 0.11 days, 95% CI −3.30 to 3.53). There was also no difference in the rate of chorioamnionitis or endometritis. Adverse neonatal outcomes including neonatal death (RR 1.60, 95% CI 0.76–3.40) were similar between the groups. The main conclusion was that the administration of progesterone was not associated with pregnancy prolongation among patients with PPROM.

SUMMARY

The limited number of publications addressing the use of tocolytics among patients with PPROM severely limits the ability to reach definitive conclusions. Recommendations from national professional societies echo these limitations. The American College of Obstetrics and Gynecology states that tocolytic agents "can be considered in preterm PPROM for steroid benefit or for maternal transport but should be used cautiously."[1] The Royal College of Obstetricians and Gynecologists concluded that because of the lack of significantly improve perinatal outcome and the potential association with an increased risk of chorioamnionitis reported by the Cochrane review, they conclude that "tocolysis in patients with PPROM is not recommended."[5]

Although the meta-analyses currently available attempt to clarify this clinical conundrum, the relatively small number of patients present even when combining all published trials still hinders drawing generalizable conclusions. In addition, several interventions known to improve perinatal outcomes such as corticosteroids were not used in many of the earlier trials. Because most adverse outcomes are rare, even at early gestational ages, the small sample sizes impede an adequate assessment of maternal-fetal benefit and risk. If we assume that the perinatal mortality rate among patients with PPROM is approximately 7.5%,[45] a trial of 2994 women equally distributed between the groups would be required to show that the use of tocolytic therapy would lead to a decrease in the rate of this adverse outcome by one-third. Therefore, it is unlikely that definitive evidence-based conclusions will be reached in the near future. Based on the review of the data currently available, below are the evidence-based conclusions that can be reached.

CLINICS CARE POINTS

- Acute (for 48 hours) use of tocolytic agents with PPROM before 34 weeks may contribute to improved neonatal outcomes
- Before viability, there is no role for the use of tocolytics in PPROM
- A short course of tocolysis in patients with PPROM before 34 weeks may be considered allowing for steroid administration or to assist with maternal transportation to an institution with a higher level of care
- There is insufficient evidence at this time to make any recommendations for the use of a short course of tocolytics from 34 to 36 weeks attempting to obtain benefit from late preterm corticosteroids
- Magnesium sulfate for neuroprotection should be used if delivery is imminent following PROM before 32 weeks

- No tocolytic agent appears to be superior to another
- Although tocolytics are associated with an increased latency period from rupture to delivery, their use may also be associated with an increased risk of intrauterine infection
- Using 17-hydroxyprogesterone caproate as an agent to prolong pregnancy in cases of PPROM appears to be ineffective
- Cases complicated by PPROM with a cerclage in place, there is insufficient evidence to make a clear recommendation on removal versus retention
- A shared decision-making approach should always be used when deciding on the risk and benefits of tocolytic agents with a patient diagnosed with PPROM

DISCLOSURE

The authors have nothing to disclose.

REFERENCES

1. Prelabor Rupture of Membranes: ACOG Practice Bulletin, Number 217. Obstet Gynecol 2020;135:e80–97.
2. Parry S, Strauss JF 3rd. Premature rupture of the fetal membranes. N Engl J Med 1998;338:663–70.
3. Goldenberg RL, Culhane JF, Iams JD, et al. Epidemiology and causes of preterm birth. Lancet 2008;371:75–84.
4. Mercer BM. Preterm premature rupture of the membranes. Obstet Gynecol 2003; 101:178–93.
5. Thomson AJ, Royal College of Obstetricians and Gynaecologists. Care of women presenting with suspected preterm prelabour rupture of membranes from 24(+0) weeks of gestation: green-top guideline no. 73. BJOG 2019;126:e152–66.
6. Yudin MH, van Schalkwyk J, Van Eyk N. No. 233-antibiotic therapy in preterm premature rupture of the membranes. J Obstet Gynaecol Can 2017;39:e207–12.
7. Melamed N, Hadar E, Ben-Haroush A, et al. Factors affecting the duration of the latency period in preterm premature rupture of membranes. J Matern Fetal Neonatal Med 2009;22:1051–6.
8. Mendez-Figueroa H, Dahlke JD, Viteri OA, et al. Neonatal and infant outcomes in twin gestations with preterm premature rupture of membranes at 24-31 weeks of gestation. Obstet Gynecol 2014;124:323–31.
9. Mercer BM. Is there a role for tocolytic therapy during conservative management of preterm premature rupture of the membranes? Clin Obstet Gynecol 2007;50: 487–96.
10. Kenyon S, Boulvain M, Neilson JP. Antibiotics for preterm rupture of membranes. Cochrane Database Syst Rev 2013;(12):CD001058.
11. Ramsey PS, Lieman JM, Brumfield CG, et al. Chorioamnionitis increases neonatal morbidity in pregnancies complicated by preterm premature rupture of membranes. Am J Obstet Gynecol 2005;192:1162–6.
12. Ananth CV, Oyelese Y, Srinivas N, et al. Preterm premature rupture of membranes, intrauterine infection, and oligohydramnios: risk factors for placental abruption. Obstet Gynecol 2004;104:71–7.
13. Major CA, de Veciana M, Lewis DF, et al. Preterm premature rupture of membranes and abruptio placentae: is there an association between these pregnancy complications? Am J Obstet Gynecol 1995;172:672–6.

14. Flenady V, Wojcieszek AM, Papatsonis DN, et al. Calcium channel blockers for inhibiting preterm labour and birth. Cochrane Database Syst Rev 2014;(6): CD002255.
15. Neilson JP, West HM, Dowswell T. Betamimetics for inhibiting preterm labour. Cochrane Database Syst Rev 2014;(2):CD004352.
16. Crowther CA, Middleton PF, Voysey M, et al. Assessing the neuroprotective benefits for babies of antenatal magnesium sulphate: an individual participant data meta-analysis. PLoS Med 2017;14:e1002398.
17. Roberts D, Brown J, Medley N, et al. Antenatal corticosteroids for accelerating fetal lung maturation for women at risk of preterm birth. Cochrane Database Syst Rev 2017;(3):CD004454.
18. Chatzakis C, Papatheodorou S, Sarafidis K, et al. Effect on perinatal outcome of prophylactic antibiotics in preterm prelabor rupture of membranes: network meta-analysis of randomized controlled trials. Ultrasound Obstet Gynecol 2020;55: 20–31.
19. Naik Gaunekar N, Raman P, Bain E, et al. Maintenance therapy with calcium channel blockers for preventing preterm birth after threatened preterm labour. Cochrane Database Syst Rev 2013;(3):CD004071.
20. van Vliet E, Dijkema GH, Schuit E, et al. Nifedipine maintenance tocolysis and perinatal outcome: an individual participant data meta-analysis. BJOG 2016; 123:1753–60.
21. Tsakiridis I, Mamopoulos A, Chalkia-Prapa EM, et al. Preterm premature rupture of membranes: a review of 3 national guidelines. Obstet Gynecol Surv 2018;73: 368–75.
22. Ramsey PS, Nuthalapaty FS, Lu G, et al. Contemporary management of preterm premature rupture of membranes (PPROM): a survey of maternal-fetal medicine providers. Am J Obstet Gynecol 2004;191:1497–502.
23. Buchanan S, Crowther C, Morris J. Preterm prelabour rupture of the membranes: a survey of current practice. Aust N Z J Obstet Gynaecol 2004;44:400–3.
24. Fortunato SJ, Welt SI, Eggleston M, et al. Prolongation of the latency period in preterm premature rupture of the membranes using prophylactic antibiotics and tocolysis. J Perinatol 1990;10:252–6.
25. Jazayeri A, Jazayeri MK, Sutkin G. Tocolysis does not improve neonatal outcome in patients with preterm rupture of membranes. Am J Perinatol 2003;20:189–93.
26. Combs CA, McCune M, Clark R, et al. Aggressive tocolysis does not prolong pregnancy or reduce neonatal morbidity after preterm premature rupture of the membranes. Am J Obstet Gynecol 2004;190:1723–8 [discussion: 8–31].
27. Kulmala L, Phupong V. Effect of terbutaline on latency period in preterm premature rupture of membranes. Gynecol Obstet Invest 2012;73:130–4.
28. Horton AL, Lai Y, Rouse DJ, et al. Effect of magnesium sulfate administration for neuroprotection on latency in women with preterm premature rupture of membranes. Am J Perinatol 2015;32:387–92.
29. Lorthe E, Goffinet F, Marret S, et al. Tocolysis after preterm premature rupture of membranes and neonatal outcome: a propensity-score analysis. Am J Obstet Gynecol 2017;217:212.e1–12.
30. Jung EJ, Byun JM, Kim YN, et al. Antenatal magnesium sulfate for both tocolysis and fetal neuroprotection in premature rupture of the membranes before 32 weeks' gestation. J Matern Fetal Neonatal Med 2018;31:1431–41.
31. Christensen KK, Ingemarsson I, Leideman T, et al. Effect of ritodrine on labor after premature rupture of the membranes. Obstet Gynecol 1980;55:187–90.

32. Levy DL, Warsof SL. Oral ritodrine and preterm premature rupture of membranes. Obstet Gynecol 1985;66:621–3.
33. Garite TJ, Keegan KA, Freeman RK, et al. A randomized trial of ritodrine tocolysis versus expectant management in patients with premature rupture of membranes at 25 to 30 weeks of gestation. Am J Obstet Gynecol 1987;157:388–93.
34. Weiner CP, Renk K, Klugman M. The therapeutic efficacy and cost-effectiveness of aggressive tocolysis for premature labor associated with premature rupture of the membranes. Am J Obstet Gynecol 1988;159:216–22.
35. Matsuda Y, Ikenoue T, Hokanishi H. Premature rupture of the membranes-aggressive versus conservative approach: effect of tocolytic and antibiotic therapy. Gynecol Obstet Invest 1993;36:102–7.
36. Dunlop P, Crowley P, Lamont R, et al. Preterm ruptured membranes, no contractions. J Obstet Gynecol 1986;7:92–6.
37. Decavalas G, Mastrogiannis D, Papadopoulos V, et al. Short-term verus long-term prophylactic tocolysis in patients with preterm premature rupture of membranes. Eur J Obstet Gynecol Reprod Biol 1995;59:143–7.
38. How HY, Cook CR, Cook VD, et al. Preterm premature rupture of membranes: aggressive tocolysis versus expectant management. J Matern Fetal Med 1998; 7:8–12.
39. Ehsanipoor RM, Shrivastava VK, Lee RM, et al. A randomized, double-masked trial of prophylactic indomethacin tocolysis versus placebo in women with premature rupture of membranes. Am J Perinatol 2011;28:473–8.
40. Galyean A, Garite TJ, Maurel K, et al. Removal versus retention of cerclage in preterm premature rupture of membranes: a randomized controlled trial. Am J Obstet Gynecol 2014;211:399.e1–7.
41. Meis PJ, Klebanoff M, Thom E, et al. Prevention of recurrent preterm delivery by 17 alpha-hydroxyprogesterone caproate. N Engl J Med 2003;348:2379–85.
42. Combs CA, Garite TJ, Maurel K, et al. 17-hydroxyprogesterone caproate for preterm rupture of the membranes: a multicenter, randomized, double-blind, placebo-controlled trial. Am J Obstet Gynecol 2015;213:364.e1–12.
43. Nijman TA, van Vliet EO, Naaktgeboren CA, et al. Nifedipine versus placebo in the treatment of preterm prelabor rupture of membranes: a randomized controlled trial: Assessment of perinatal outcome by use of tocolysis in early labor-APOSTEL IV trial. Eur J Obstet Gynecol Reprod Biol 2016;205:79–84.
44. Ohlsson A. Treatments of preterm premature rupture of the membranes: a meta-analysis. Am J Obstet Gynecol 1989;160:890–906.
45. Mackeen AD, Seibel-Seamon J, Muhammad J, et al. Tocolytics for preterm premature rupture of membranes. Cochrane Database Syst Rev 2014;(2):CD007062.
46. Quist-Nelson J, Parker P, Mokhtari N, et al. Progestogens in singleton gestations with preterm prelabor rupture of membranes: a systematic review and metaanalysis of randomized controlled trials. Am J Obstet Gynecol 2018;219: 346–355 e2.

Use of Antenatal Corticosteroids in Preterm Prelabor Rupture of Membranes

Ashley N. Battarbee, MD, MSCR

KEYWORDS

- Antenatal corticosteroids • Betamethasone
- Preterm prelabor rupture of membranes • Respiratory distress syndrome
- Neonatal mortality

KEY POINTS

- Antenatal corticosteroids reduce the risk of neonatal morbidity and mortality among women with preterm prelabor rupture of membranes (PPROM).
- There is no increased risk of maternal or neonatal infection after administration of antenatal corticosteroids even after PPROM.
- There is insufficient evidence to recommend for or against a single rescue course of antenatal corticosteroids in women with PPROM.

INTRODUCTION

Antenatal corticosteroids are among the most important interventions to prevent neonatal morbidity and mortality associated with preterm birth. The beneficial effects of corticosteroids were first discovered in the late 1960s during experiments of parturition using a sheep model. Graham Liggins[1] discovered that exogenous administration of large doses of corticosteroids intended to induce labor resulted in preterm lambs who had structurally more mature lungs and survived longer compared with controls.[1] He subsequently collaborated with pediatrician Ross Howie, and in 1972 they published the first randomized clinical trial in humans, which demonstrated that two 12-mg intramuscular injections of betamethasone reduced the frequency of respiratory distress syndrome compared with placebo (25.8% vs 9.0%, $P = .003$).[2] Furthermore, antenatally administered betamethasone reduced the frequency of early neonatal mortality (15.0% vs 3.2%, $P = .01$). Although this study offered promising results, the use of antenatal corticosteroids in clinical practice was not universally adopted due to unwarranted fears about potential adverse side

Department of Obstetrics and Gynecology, Center for Women's Reproductive Health, University of Alabama at Birmingham, 1700 6th Avenue South, Women & Infants Center Room 10270, Birmingham, AL 35233, USA
E-mail address: anbattarbee@uabmc.edu

Obstet Gynecol Clin N Am 47 (2020) 587–594
https://doi.org/10.1016/j.ogc.2020.08.004
0889-8545/20/© 2020 Elsevier Inc. All rights reserved.

effects. Countless clinical trials aimed at confirming the respiratory benefits and investigating possible adverse effects continued through the 1990s until a systematic review and meta-analysis concluded that there was irrefutable evidence of the efficacy and safety of antenatal corticosteroids. This meta-analysis of 15 randomized controlled trials demonstrated a reduction in respiratory distress syndrome (typical odds ratio [OR] 0.5, 95% confidence interval [CI] 0.4–0.6) as well as reductions in periventricular hemorrhage, necrotizing enterocolitis, and neonatal mortality without any significant increase in maternal infection.[3] The results of this meta-analysis and other pertinent publications were reviewed by the National Institutes of Health (NIH) consensus panel including 16 experts from neonatology, obstetrics, family medicine, behavioral medicine, psychology, biostatistics, and the public. The panel concluded that antenatal corticosteroid therapy is indicated for women at risk for premature delivery with few exceptions and will result in a substantial decrease in neonatal morbidity and mortality.[4] With the ensuing endorsement from other national organizations, such as the American College of Obstetricians and Gynecologists (ACOG), the use of antenatal corticosteroids in clinical practice rose dramatically. The beneficial effects of antenatal corticosteroids continue to be appreciated since that time, with the most recent Cochrane review of 30 randomized controlled trials including 8158 infants demonstrating a reduction in neonatal morbidity and mortality with no significant maternal or neonatal risks (**Table 1**).[5]

ANTENATAL CORTICOSTEROIDS REDUCE NEONATAL MORBIDITY AND MORTALITY AFTER PRETERM PRELABOR RUPTURE OF MEMBRANES WITHOUT INCREASING THE RISK OF MATERNAL OR NEONATAL INFECTION

Although the original trial by Liggins and Howie[2] in 1972 demonstrated a reduction in neonatal respiratory distress syndrome among women with preterm prelabor rupture of membranes (PPROM) (typical OR 0.44, 95% CI 0.32–0.60) and no increased risk of infection overall, there has been extensive debate about the utility of antenatal corticosteroids in this population. Initially, some small studies noted an increase in maternal infection and prolonged neonatal hospitalization and questioned the efficacy

Table 1
Summary of outcomes among women at high risk of preterm birth who received antenatal corticosteroids versus placebo or no treatment from the 2017 Cochrane Review[5]

Maternal and Neonatal Outcomes	Average Relative Risk (95% Confidence Interval)	Number of Participants (Studies)
Perinatal death	0.72 (0.58–0.89)	6279 (15 RCTs)
Neonatal death	0.69 (0.59–0.81)	7188 (22 RCTs)
Respiratory distress syndrome	0.66 (0.56–0.77)	7764 (28 RCTs)
Intraventricular hemorrhage	0.55 (0.32–0.78)	6093 (16 RCTs)
Necrotizing enterocolitis	0.50 (0.32–0.78)	4702 (10 RCTs)
Neonatal mechanical ventilation	0.68 (0.56–0.84)	1368 (9 RCTs)
Systemic infection within first 48 h of life	0.60 (0.41–0.88)	1753 (8 RCTs)
Chorioamnionitis	0.83 (0.66–1.06)	5546 (15 RCTs)
Endometritis	1.20 (0.87–1.63)	4030 (10 RCTs)

Abbreviation: RCTs, randomized controlled trials.

of antenatal corticosteroids in reducing respiratory morbidity in women with PPROM. For example, in a randomized controlled trial of 73 women with PPROM, there was an increased incidence of postpartum febrile morbidity and no reduction in respiratory distress syndrome in the intervention group compared with controls. However, this 1985 study was limited by small sample size and use of hydrocortisone rather than betamethasone or dexamethasone for the intervention group.[6] A slightly larger randomized controlled trial of 160 women with PPROM also found an increased risk for maternal endometritis after treatment with corticosteroids, but the women who were randomized to corticosteroids were delivered after 48 hours, whereas women who were randomized to the control group were managed expectantly until development of chorioamnionitis or another indication for delivery.[7] It is also important to note that both of these early studies were performed before the discovery and incorporation of latency antibiotics into the management of PPROM.[8] However, due to the potential increased risk of infection and relatively lower rates of respiratory immaturity at later gestational ages, the NIH Consensus panel initially recommended use of antenatal corticosteroids only up to 30 to 32 weeks' gestation in women with PPROM.[4]

The best current evidence shows that antenatal corticosteroids are effective at reducing neonatal morbidity and mortality without an increased risk of maternal or neonatal infection in the setting of PPROM. In a meta-analysis of 15 randomized controlled trials involving more than 1400 women with PPROM, antenatal corticosteroids reduced the risks of respiratory distress syndrome (relative risk [RR] 0.56, 95% CI 0.31–0.70) and intraventricular hemorrhage (RR 0.47, 95% CI 0.05–0.82) with a trend toward reduction in neonatal death (RR 0.68, 95% CI 0.43–1.07) compared with controls.[9] There did not appear to be any increase in maternal infection (RR 0.86, 95% CI 0.61–1.20) or neonatal infection (RR 1.05, 95% CI 0.66–1.68). In a subsequent meta-analysis including 17 randomized controlled trials and more than 1900 women with PPROM, antenatal corticosteroids were again found to reduce the risk of respiratory distress syndrome (RR 0.81, 95% CI 0.67–0.98) and grade III and IV intraventricular hemorrhage (RR 0.49, 95% CI 0.25–0.96) with no significant increase in neonatal sepsis or maternal chorioamnionitis. Similarly, the most recent Cochrane review found no significant differences in the effect of antenatal corticosteroids among the subgroup of women with PPROM rather than other indications for preterm birth (**Table 2**).[5] Compared with placebo or no treatment, antenatal corticosteroids reduced

Table 2
Summary of outcomes among the subgroup of women with preterm prelabor rupture of membranes who received antenatal corticosteroids versus placebo or no treatment from the 2017 Cochrane Review[5]

Maternal and Neonatal Outcomes	Average Relative Risk (95% Confidence Interval)	Number of Participants (Studies)
Perinatal death	0.59 (0.39–0.90)	733 (4 RCTs)
Neonatal death	0.61 (0.46–0.83)	1024 (8 RCTs)
Respiratory distress syndrome	0.70 (0.55–0.90)	1129 (12 RCTs)
Intraventricular hemorrhage	0.47 (0.28–0.79)	895 (5 RCTs)
Chorioamnionitis	0.98 (0.69–1.40)	959 (7 RCTs)
Endometritis	1.02 (0.35–2.97)	477 (4 RCTs)

Abbreviation: RCTs, randomized controlled trials.

the risk of respiratory distress syndrome, intraventricular hemorrhage, and neonatal death without an increase in chorioamnionitis or endometritis. Thus, the most recent recommendations from ACOG do not restrict antenatal corticosteroids to only women with PPROM less than 30 to 32 weeks' gestation.[10,11]

ANTENATAL CORTICOSTEROIDS AFTER PRETERM PRELABOR RUPTURE OF MEMBRANES AT DIFFERENT GESTATIONAL AGES

Neonatal morbidity and mortality are inversely related to gestational age at birth and thus the potential benefit of antenatal corticosteroids should be the greatest at early gestational ages but may wane at later gestational ages. However, the effect of antenatal corticosteroids at periviable gestational ages has been debated, as resuscitation of these neonates is often limited given extremely low birthweight and only rudimentary lung development. In a prospective cohort study of 10,541 neonates born at 22 to 25 weeks' gestation, antenatal corticosteroids reduced the risk of death of neurodevelopmental impairment at 18 to 22 months of life.[12] This reduction was significant among neonates born at 23, 24, and 25 weeks' gestation, but not among those born at 22 weeks' gestation (**Fig. 1**). Similarly, analysis of prospectively collected data on 11,022 infants born at 22 0/7 to 28 6/7 weeks' gestation showed that antenatal corticosteroids reduced neonatal mortality at 23 to 27 weeks' gestation, but did not reach statistical significance among the subgroup of neonates born at 22 weeks' gestation.[13] Although it is possible that no effect was seen among the subgroup of infants born at 22 weeks simply due to smaller sample size and limited power, ACOG currently does not recommend consideration of antenatal corticosteroid administration until 23 0/7 weeks' gestation.[10,11,14] It is also important to note that although

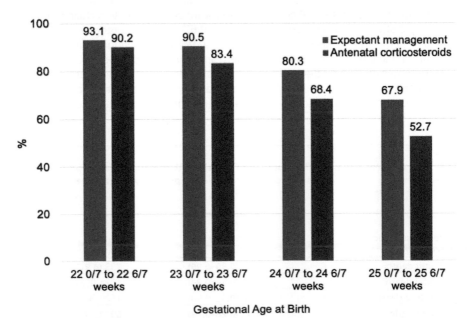

Fig. 1. Death and neurodevelopmental impairment by antenatal corticosteroid exposure among periviable births. (*Data from* Carlo WA, McDonald SA, Fanaroff AA, et al. Association of antenatal corticosteroids with mortality and neurodevelopmental outcomes among infants born at 22 to 25 weeks' gestation. Obstet Gynecol Surv. 2012;67(4):215-217.)

neonates who delivered after PPROM were included in both of these cohorts, there were no subgroup analyses performed to evaluate the effect of antenatal corticosteroids in this specific population.

On the other end of the gestational age spectrum, there are a few studies that address the effect of antenatal corticosteroids specifically among women with PPROM. In a retrospective cohort study of 191 women with PPROM at 32 0/7 to 33 6/7 weeks' gestation antenatal corticosteroids did not appear to increase the risk of chorioamnionitis, compared to no antenatal corticosteroids (12.8% vs 10.0%, p=0.43), but also did not appear to reduce the risk of respiratory distress syndrome (33.6% vs 38.5%, p=0.57).[15] The main limitation of this study is small sample size with unequal distribution of women who received antenatal corticosteroids (n = 150) and did not receive antenatal corticosteroids (n = 41). This sample size only provided 80% power to detect a RR ≥3.0 for chorioamnionitis (≥30.2% chorioamnionitis in antenatal corticosteroid group) and RR ≤0.45 for respiratory distress syndrome (≤17.3% respiratory distress syndrome in antenatal corticosteroid group). Thus, it is not surprising that the investigators did not see a reduction in respiratory distress syndrome, as the Cochrane review demonstrates that antenatal corticosteroids only reduce respiratory distress syndrome by RR 0.66 in an unselected population and RR 0.70 in women with PPROM.[16]

In a recent randomized controlled trial of women with threatened late preterm birth between 34 0/7 and 36 6/7 weeks' gestation, antenatal betamethasone was found to reduce the frequency of composite respiratory morbidity (11.6% vs 14.4%; RR 0.80, 95% CI 0.66–0.90) and severe respiratory complications (8.1% vs 12.1%; RR 0.67, 95% CI 0.53–0.84).[17] Among this cohort of 2831 women, 620 (22%) women had PPROM. PPROM compared with other indications for trial entry was evaluated as one of the prespecified subgroup analyses to determine if there was a differential effect of antenatal betamethasone on composite respiratory morbidity or severe respiratory complications.[18] There was no evidence of interaction between indication for trial entry (preterm labor, preterm premature rupture of membranes, or other obstetric or medical indication for preterm delivery) and the composite respiratory morbidity (P = .083) or severe respiratory complication (P = .38). The lack of significant interaction between indication for trial entry and the effect of betamethasone on the primary outcome indicates that the effect of late preterm betamethasone is not any different among women with PPROM compared to women with another indication for late preterm delivery. Based on these findings and lack of evidence of harm, ACOG recommends a single course of antenatal corticosteroids between 34 0/7 and 36 5/7 weeks' gestation if they have not received a prior course of corticosteroids.

REPEAT COURSES OF ANTENATAL CORTICOSTEROIDS AFTER PRETERM PRELABOR RUPTURE OF MEMBRANES

Because a single 48-hour course of antenatal corticosteroids was effective at reducing preterm neonatal morbidity and mortality, it was initially thought that multiple courses among women who remained undelivered could be even better. To study that hypothesis, a randomized double-blind, placebo-controlled trial enrolled 437 women with threatened preterm birth who had completed a single course of antenatal corticosteroids before 30 weeks and at least 14 days before enrollment and randomized them to receive a repeat or "rescue" course of antenatal corticosteroids or identical-appearing placebo.[19] A single "rescue" course of antenatal corticosteroids reduced composite neonatal morbidity (OR 0.45, 95% CI 0.27–0.75). However, women with PPROM were excluded from this study and thus the effect in this population remained unknown.

Subsequent studies evaluating the effect of a "rescue" course of antenatal cortico-steroids among women with PPROM are limited by small sample size. In a secondary analysis of 1641 women with PPROM (1496 received 1 course and 145 received a single repeat course of ACS), there was no reduction in respiratory distress syndrome (48.9% vs 54.5%, $P = .20$). Although there was no evidence of benefit, there was also no evidence of harm with similar frequencies of chorioamnionitis (12.0% vs 11.0%, $P = .72$) and neonatal sepsis (16.2% vs 17.2%, $P = .76$) in both groups. The major limitations of this study include lack of information about timing of antenatal corticosteroid administration relative to delivery and small sample size with limited ability to detect small differences between groups. ACOG acknowledges the lack of sufficient evidence to make a recommendation about the use of a rescue course of antenatal corticosteroids but does provide guidelines for use if it is pursued. ACOG states that the rescue course should not be given unless at least 7 to 14 days have elapsed since the prior course and the patient is currently at less than 34 weeks' gestation with high risk of preterm birth within the next 7 days.[10,11]

Multiple rescue courses of antenatal corticosteroids are not recommended as there is evidence of reduction in birthweight and head circumference at birth in unselected populations. Specifically among women with PPROM, there is evidence that multiple courses of antenatal corticosteroids increase the risk of early-onset neonatal sepsis, chorioamnionitis, and endometritis.[20,21] For these reasons, more than 1 rescue course of antenatal corticosteroids is not recommended for women with PPROM or threatened preterm birth for any other indication.[11]

SUMMARY AND FUTURE DIRECTIONS

In summary, there is evidence to support administration of a single course of antenatal corticosteroids for pregnant women with PPROM between 24 0/7 and 33 6/7 weeks' gestation. ACOG states that antenatal corticosteroids may also be considered for pregnant women starting at 23 0/7 weeks' gestation and between 34 0/7 and 36 5/7 weeks' gestation if they have not received a prior course of corticosteroids based on limited data. Currently there is insufficient evidence to recommend for or against administration of a single rescue course of antenatal corticosteroids after PPROM. ACOG acknowledges that it is controversial, but they cite the secondary analysis showing no increased risk of harm and state that a single rescue course may be provided as early as 7 days after the prior course for women less than 34 0/7 who are at risk of delivery within 7 days. Further studies of women with PPROM are needed to investigate the effect of antenatal corticosteroids at less than 23 weeks' gestation and a single rescue course of antenatal corticosteroids at later gestational ages. Antenatal corticosteroids are one of the greatest discoveries to prevent neonatal morbidity and mortality associated with preterm birth and they should not be withheld in the setting of PPROM.

CLINICS CARE POINTS

- A course of antenatal corticosteroids (i.e. two doses of 12mg betamethasone given 24 hours apart) should be administered to women with PPROM to reduce the risk of neonatal morbidity and mortality.
- A single course of antenatal corticosteroids does not increase the risk for maternal or neonatal infection.
- Administration of a single rescue course of antenatal corticosteroids may be considered as there is currently not overwhelming evidence of benefit or of harm in women with PPROM.

DISCLOSURE

The author has nothing to disclose.

REFERENCES

1. Liggins GC. Premature delivery of foetal lambs infused with glucocorticoids. J Endocrinol 1969;45(4):515–23.
2. Liggins GC, Howie RN. A controlled trial of antepartum glucocorticoid treatment for prevention of the respiratory distress syndrome in premature infants. Pediatrics 1972;50(4):515–25.
3. Crowley PA. Antenatal corticosteroid therapy: a meta-analysis of the randomized trials, 1972 to 1994. Am J Obstet Gynecol 1995;173(1):322–35.
4. Effect of corticosteroids for fetal maturation on perinatal outcomes. NIH Consensus Statement. JAMA 1995;273(5):413–8.
5. Roberts D, Brown J, Medley N, et al. Antenatal corticosteroids for accelerating fetal lung maturation for women at risk of preterm birth. Cochrane Database Syst Rev 2017;(3):CD004454.
6. Iams JD, Talbert ML, Barrows H, et al. Management of preterm prematurely ruptured membranes: a prospective randomized comparison of observation versus use of steroids and timed delivery. Am J Obstet Gynecol 1985;151(1):32–8.
7. Garite TJ, Freeman RK, Linzey EM. Prospective randomized study of corticosteroids in the management of premature rupture of the membranes and the premature gestation. Am J Obstet Gynecol 1981;141(5):508–15.
8. Mercer BM, Egarter C, Leitich H. Antibiotic treatment for preterm premature rupture of membranes [9]. Am J Obstet Gynecol 1996;175(3 I):755–6.
9. Harding JE, Pang JM, Knight DB, et al. Do antenatal corticosteroids help in the setting of preterm rupture of membranes? Am J Obstet Gynecol 2001;184(2):131–9.
10. American College of Obstetricians and Gynecologists. Prelabor rupture of membranes. ACOG Practice Bulletin No. 217. Obstet Gynecol 2020;135(3):e80–97.
11. Committee on Obstetric Practice. Committee Opinion No. 713. Obstet Gynecol 2017;130(2):e102–9.
12. Carlo WA, McDonald SA, Fanaroff AA, et al. Association of antenatal corticosteroids with mortality and neurodevelopmental outcomes among infants born at 22 to 25 weeks' gestation. Obstet Gynecol Surv 2012;67(4):215–7.
13. Travers CP, Carlo WA, McDonald SA, et al. Mortality and pulmonary outcomes of extremely preterm infants exposed to antenatal corticosteroids. Am J Obstet Gynecol 2018;218(1):130.e1–13.
14. Periviable birth. Obstetric Care Consensus No. 6. American College of Obstetricians and Gynecologists. Obstet Gynecol 2017;130(4):926–8.
15. Sheibani L, Fong A, Henry DE, et al. Maternal and neonatal outcomes after antenatal corticosteroid administration for PPROM at 32 to 33 6/7 weeks gestational age*. J Matern Fetal Neonatal Med 2017;30(14):1676–80.
16. Roberts D, Brown J, Medley NDS. Antenatal corticosteroids for accelerating fetal lung maturation for women at risk of preterm birth. Obstet Gynecol 2007;109(1):189–90.
17. Gyamfi-Bannerman C, Thom EA, Blackwell SC, et al. Antenatal betamethasone for women at risk for late preterm delivery. N Engl J Med 2016;374(14):1311–20.
18. Gyamfi-Bannerman C, Thom EA, Blackwell SC, et al. Supplementary appendix of antenatal betamethasone for women at risk for late preterm delivery. N Engl J Med 2016;374:1311–20.

19. Garite TJ, Kurtzman J, Maurel K, et al. Impact of a "rescue course" of antenatal corticosteroids: a multicenter randomized placebo-controlled trial. Am J Obstet Gynecol 2009;200(3):248.e1–9.
20. Vermillion ST, Soper DE, Chasedunn-Roark J. Neonatal sepsis after betamethasone administration to patients with preterm premature rupture of membranes. Am J Obstet Gynecol 1999;181(2):320–7.
21. Yang S, Choi S, Roh C, et al. Multiple courses of antenatal corticosteroid therapy in patients with preterm premature rupture of membranes. J Perinat Med 2004; 32(1):42–8.

Antibiotics for Prophylaxis in the Setting of Preterm Prelabor Rupture of Membranes

Sarah Dotters-Katz, MD, MMHPE

KEYWORDS

- PPROM • Latency • Antibiotics • Preterm prelabor rupture of membranes

KEY POINTS

- The use of antibiotics in the setting of preterm prelabor rupture of membranes decreases both maternal and neonatal infection rates and increases latency until delivery.
- Although multiple regimens have been studied, the current recommended regimen is ampicillin 2 g intravenously (IV) every 6 hours × 48 hours, then amoxicillin 250 mg orally (PO) every 8 hours × 5 days AND erythromycin 250 mg IV every 6 hours × 48 hours, then erythromycin 333 mg PO every 8 hours × 5 days.
- Latency antibiotics are recommended for use in PPROM after viability until 33 weeks and 6 days of gestational age in the setting on singletons and multiple gestations.

BACKGROUND

Preterm prelabor rupture of membranes (PPROM) occurs in 3% to 4% of all pregnancies, and is the cause of 25% to 30% of all preterm births.[1] Although the exact cause of PPROM is unknown, and believed to be multifactorial, infection and inflammation are thought to have a major role. Although infection is often implicated in causality, in other cases it occurs after membrane rupture. It is believed that pathologic bacteria produce proteases, collagenases, and/or mucinases that impair membrane integrity, initiate inflammatory cascades, and ultimately lead to rupture.[2] In cases of secondary infection, the bacteria are thought to ascend from the vagina and lead to intra-amniotic infection and/or fetal infection.

Whether causal or secondary, infection has been linked to adverse neonatal outcomes, further exacerbating the risk of prematurity itself. Neurologic damage, including cerebral palsy, chronic lung disease, intraventricular hemorrhage, neonatal sepsis, necrotizing enterocolitis (NEC) and death have all been associated with intra-amniotic infection.[3] Though the impacts on the fetus can be dire, maternal

Department of Obstetrics and Gynecology, Duke University, Duke University School of Medicine, 2608 Erwin Road, Suite 210, Durham, NC 27705, USA
E-mail address: sd132@duke.edu
Twitter: @sarahdk8383 (S.D.-K.)

Obstet Gynecol Clin N Am 47 (2020) 595–603
https://doi.org/10.1016/j.ogc.2020.08.005
0889-8545/20/© 2020 Elsevier Inc. All rights reserved.

implications of infection are also potentially quite morbid. Maternal risks of antepartum intra-amniotic infection include sepsis, endometritis, postpartum hemorrhage, and in rare cases result in intensive care unit admission and even death.[4] Thus, for both maternal and fetal benefit, antibiotics have long been considered an integral part of the management of PPROM.

It is also important to note that although antibiotics play a critical role in the management of women with PPROM, they are not the only integral aspects. Women who present with PPROM between viability and 33 weeks and 6 days should be given corticosteroids for fetal lung maturity.[5] Corticosteroids in this context is not believed to negatively impact the risk of infectious morbidity. For women who rupture membranes between viability and 32 weeks, the use of magnesium for neuroprotection is also recommended.[5] These topics are further discussed in other sections, but are important to recognize as other critical management aspects for these patients. Finally, for the purposes of this article, unless otherwise specified, PPROM recommendations regarding latency antibiotics refer to cases in which membrane rupture occurs after viability and before 34 weeks and 0 days.

WHAT BACTERIA ARE WE TREATING?

The ultimate goal of antibiotics in the setting of PPROM is to avoid maternal and fetal infection, thereby prolonging pregnancy. A common pathogen isolated in all cases of intra-amniotic infection, as well as specifically in the setting of intra-amniotic infection in the setting of PPROM is *Ureaplasma urealyticum*.[6,7] Other common pathogens include *Mycoplasma hominis,* Streptococcal species, and Staphylococcal species.[6–8] Other studies have noted that enteric gram-negative flora and anaerobes are also common in these polymicrobial infections.[8,9] Given the true polymicrobial nature of these infections, the antibiotic choice should thoughtfully cover this wide array of organisms.

WHAT IS THE EVIDENCE BEHIND THE USE OF ANTIBIOTICS AT ALL IN THE SETTING OF PRETERM PRELABOR RUPTURE OF MEMBRANES?

The use of antibiotics for PPROM is truly evidence-based medicine. A recent Cochrane review on this topic analyzed the existing articles and found multiple improved outcomes. The use of antibiotics compared with no antibiotics for PPROM resulted in 33% reduction in neonatal infection among 12 trials involving 1680 infants.[10] In this analysis, no significant differences in respiratory distress syndrome, NEC, or the need for mechanical ventilation was identified. However, among 6289 infants in 12 trials with head ultrasound follow-up, there was a 19% decrease in abnormal cerebral ultrasounds at hospital discharge with antibiotic treatment.[10] Similarly, in 3 trials that reported neonatal length of stay, including 225 infants, the mean length of stay was 5 days shorter in infants born to mothers receiving antibiotics.[10] The ORACLE study followed children out to 7 years. Among the 3171 children, no difference in functional impairment between children born to mothers receiving antibiotics and those born to women receiving placebo was identified.[10,11]

The Cochran review also evaluated maternal outcomes. Among 1559 women in 11 trials, there were lower rates of chorioamnionitis (Relative risk 66%, 95% confidence interval [CI] 0.46–0.96).[10] No differences in rates of cesarean delivery were noted. Women receiving antibiotics were shown to have higher latency rates at 48 hours and 7 days. No maternal mortality was reported in any of the included studies.

Thus, based on this meta-analysis, there is clear benefit to the mother and the neonate with the use antibiotics in the setting of PPROM.

WHAT ANTIBIOTICS ARE RECOMMENDED FOR THE TREATMENT OF PRETERM PRELABOR RUPTURE OF MEMBRANES?

The suspicion that infection and inflammation play a role in the pathogenesis and natural history of PPROM, led clinicians to prescribe a variety of antibiotics for this indication for more than 30 years. However, as more studies have been performed, the specific regimens and durations have evolved. This next section will outline the evolution of the recommendations.

In 1997, Mercer and colleagues[12] published the landmark trial that standardized the recommendation for treatment. This multicenter randomized double-blind placebo-controlled trial randomized 614 women with intravenous ampicillin (2 g every 6 hours) and erythromycin (250 mg every 8 hours) for 48 hours, followed by 5 days of oral amoxicillin (250 mg every 8 hours) and erythromycin (333 mg every 8 hours) versus placebo. In this study, the primary outcome of neonatal morbidity and mortality was less common in the antibiotic group, as was respiratory distress, stage 2 or 3 NEC, neonatal sepsis, and neonatal pneumonia. Perhaps the most significant finding of this study was the significant pregnancy prolongation seen among Group Beta Strep (GBS) negative women who received antibiotics. Their median prolongation was 6.1 days compared with only 2.9 days in the placebo group. Plus, the treatment group was more likely to be pregnant at 2 days after rupture, 7 days, 14 days, and 21 days compared with control. Mercer and colleagues[12] used the phrase, "improvement in latency" to describe this finding. Thus, many clinicians refer to the specific use of antibiotics after PPROM as "latency antibiotics." For the remainder of this article, we also use this phrase.

Based on this trial, the regimen of ampicillin and erythromycin became the standard of care for treatment of women with PPROM. Since that time, many studies comparing alternative regimens have been performed. A recent Cochrane review performed subgroup comparisons between multiple regimens, finding no differences in maternal morbidities or composite neonatal morbidities, but did note that beta lactamase inhibiting antibiotics were associated with increased rates of NEC (RR 4.72, 95% CI 1.57–14.23).[10] Kenyon and colleagues[13] randomized 2415 women with PPROM to co-amoxiclav (combination of amoxicillin and clavulanic acid) with erythromycin. Although delivery within 48 hours was lower in the co-amoxiclav group, rates of NEC were 4 times higher among women who received co-amoxiclav alone compared with placebo, and 2.5-fold higher among women who received any co-amoxiclav to no co-amoxiclav.[13] Based on these findings, the investigators recommend against the use of co-amoxiclav for latency in the setting of PPROM.

The duration of treatment is another topic that is quite variable across studies. Before the trial of Mercer and colleagues[12] in 1997, it was not uncommon for randomized trials to continue antibiotics from the time of rupture until delivery,[14–18] although other studies had treatment regimens that defined treatment length from 1 day,[19] to 3 days,[20] to 7 days.[21,22] The study by Kenyon and colleagues[13] compared erythromycin with co-amoxiclav up to 10 days or until delivery. Two trials have compared 3 versus 7 days of treatment. Lewis and colleagues[23] randomized 84 women to either 3 or 7 days of ampicillin-sulbactam, and found no differences in latency. Similarly, Segel and colleagues[24] randomized 48 women to 3 or 7 days of ampicillin, and also saw no difference in latency. In the Cochrane review, these data were merged, and outcomes did not differ.[12] The current recommendation from American College of Obstetricians and Gynecologists (ACOG) is for a 7-day course of antibiotics.

Though the original studies were done with erythromycin, this medication has been associated with an unfavorable side-effect profile. The most common side effects are gastrointestinal, specifically nausea, vomiting, and diarrhea. In contrast, azithromycin is within the same family, but has a much more benign side-effect profile. Pierson and colleagues[25] retrospectively assessed latency differences among 75 women who received erythromycin and 93 who received azithromycin, showing no difference in latency, nor intra-amniotic infection or neonatal sepsis. Another more recent retrospective cohort compared 132 women who received erythromycin and 243 who received azithromycin, also showing no difference in latency, maternal or neonatal outcomes.[26] A recent cost analysis showed azithromycin to be cost saving compared to erythromycin. Currently, the ACOG recommends erythromycin, but recognizes that many centers substitute azithromycin as a reasonable alternative.[5] Current ACOG recommendations for antibiotic choice, dosing, and duration are found in **Table 1**.

GESTATIONAL AGE VARIATIONS

For women with PPROM after viability but before 34 weeks and 0 days, ACOG currently recommends antibiotics for improved latency.[5] Because viability is variably defined by institution, the investigators have elected to use this term instead of noting a lower limit of gestational age. However, it should be noted that ACOG uses 24/0 in the most recent guideline.[27] At centers where neonatal resuscitation is offered before this gestational age, it is very reasonable to recommend latency antibiotics in the setting of membrane rupture starting when rupture occurs at that gestational age.

Quite recently, data have emerged suggesting improved neonatal outcomes with shorter neonatal length of stay in the setting of expectant management for PPROM occurring after 34 weeks, until term, defined as 37 weeks.[28] In this trial, no standardized protocol regarding latency antibiotics was reported. A more recent meta-analysis showed similar results with regard to neonatal outcomes.[29] Using participant-level data, the investigators also performed a subgroup analysis by receipt of latency antibiotics, which showed no differences in neonatal outcomes by antibiotic receipt.[29] Thus, ACOG currently does not recommend the use of latency antibiotics when PPROM is managed expectantly after 34 weeks.[5]

The use of antibiotics for pregnancy latency in the setting of previable PPROM is less clear cut and discussed elsewhere in this series.

Table 1 Antibiotic choice, dosing, and frequency based on PCN allergy status	
Antibiotic Recommendations	
No PCN allergy:	Ampicillin 2g IV every 6 h × 48 h, then amoxicillin 250 mg PO every 8 h × 5 d AND erythromycin 250 mg IV every 6 h × 48 h, then erythromycin 333 mg PO every 8 h × 5 d[a]
Mild PCN allergy:	Cefazolin 1g IV every 8 h for 48 h, then cephalexin 500 mg PO every 6 h for 5 d Erythromycin 250 mg IV every 6 h × 48 h, then erythromycin 333 mg PO every 8 h × 5 d[a]
Severe PCN allergy:	Clindamycin 900 mg IV every 8 h AND gentamicin 5 mg/kg actual body weight IV daily for 48 h, then clindamycin 300 mg PO every 8 h for 5 d Erythromycin 250 mg IV every 6 h × 48 h, then erythromycin 333 mg PO every 8 h × 5 d[a]

Abbreviations: IV, intravenous; PCN, penicillin; PO, oral.
[a] Azithromycin is an acceptable alternative.

SPECIAL CONSIDERATIONS: MULTIPLE GESTATIONS

PPROM occurs more frequently in multiple gestations than in singleton pregnancies, and retrospective data suggest that latency tends to be shorter in multiple gestations.[30,31] No studies specific to the use of antibiotics for pregnancy latency in twins or higher-order multiples specifically have been performed. Twin gestations were included in many of the original studies, specifically Mercer and colleagues[12] and Kenyon and colleagues.[32] Thus, most providers manage multiple gestations with PPROM similarly to singletons with regard to latency antibiotics.

This is also true with regard to multiple gestations who have previable PPROM, which is more also common than in singletons. One retrospective study looked specifically at the impact of latency antibiotics in 30 twin gestations with previable PPROM.[33] This study did not show a difference in median latency, or in maternal or neonatal outcomes. However, given that this is a small, single-center study, in the setting of previable PPROM in multiple gestation, it remains prudent to consider each case in the setting of extensive counseling and shared decision making.[5,34,35]

SPECIAL CONSIDERATIONS: PENICILLIN ALLERGY OR MACROLIDE ALLERGY

What antibiotic regimen to use for women with PPROM with penicillin (PCN) allergy always poses a challenging question when this scenario arises in the clinical setting. Although data specific to PPROM do not exist, recommendations have been extrapolated from other clinical scenarios where this conundrum arises in obstetrics. In these cases, antibiotic regimens should be 7 days' total duration, with 2 days of intravenous therapy and 5 days of oral therapy. For women with a mild allergy, that is, low risk for anaphylaxis, first-generation and second-generation cephalosporins are thought to be safe.[36] Thus, cefazolin 1 g intravenous every 8 hours for 48 hours, then cephalexin 500 mg orally every 6 hours for 5 days is recommended. These women should receive the standard macrolide for 7 days as well. Women who are high risk for anaphylaxis should receive clindamycin 900 mg every 8 hours and gentamicin 5 mg/kg actual body weight intravenously daily for 48 hours, followed by clindamycin alone, 300 mg orally every 8 hours for 5 days.[36] These women should also receive the standard macrolide for 7 days.

Data regarding efficacy of these regimens are limited. One retrospective study, which included 128 women who did not receive a beta-lactam (PCN or cephalosporin) -containing regimen, that is, high-risk allergies, were compared with 821 who received a beta-lactam–containing regimen.[37] In this study, latency did not differ. However, endometritis was higher in the non–beta-lactam group. This study also found higher rates of NEC in the beta-lactam group and higher rates of bronchopulmonary dysplasia in the non–beta-lactam group, although adjusted analyses were not performed on these outcomes. Although this study raises many questions, it also highlights the importance of PCN allergy testing among women with PCN allergies.

Macrolide allergies are much less common than PCN allergies. It is also important to assess if this is an intolerance or a true medication allergy. In these cases, there are not clear alternative regimens with proven efficacy. Providers can consider giving only the ampicillin portion of the regimen.

SPECIAL CONSIDERATIONS: KNOWN GROUP BETA STREP NEGATIVE AT TIME OF PRETERM PRELABOR RUPTURE OF MEMBRANES

For women who present with PPROM and who have an unknown GBS status, GBS testing should be performed, and treatment with ampicillin should occur. If the GBS culture returns negative before the end of the recommended 7-day course, it is reasonable to complete the antibiotic course.[38] Retesting should occur every 5 weeks if the patient remains pregnant.

Women who have had a positive GBS culture within the past 5 weeks or who have had a positive urine culture for GBS should also be treated with ampicillin. Repeat testing does not need to occur in these cases.

In rare cases, women presenting with PPROM will have had a GBS test in the few weeks prior for preterm labor or other unrelated reason. In cases in which the culture is negative, and the patient subsequently presents with PPROM, no guidance exists to the appropriate course of action. Given the low cost and low-risk profile, in addition to the benefit seen in the GBS-negative arm in the trial of Mercer and colleagues,[12] most providers would still include ampicillin and amoxicillin in the latency regimen.[12]

SPECIAL CONSIDERATIONS: ONSET OF LABOR WITHIN 7 DAYS OF RUPTURE?

Approximately 50% of women will labor within 7 days of rupture.[12] Many of these women will be on latency antibiotics when labor ensues. In these cases, GBS prophylaxis should continue for women who are GBS unknown and GBS positive. Although no specific guidance exists, it is reasonable to continue the macrolide as well. Once the patient delivers, all antibiotics can be stopped, unless another obstetric indication for postpartum antibiotics exists. Evaluation for chorioamnionitis should be performed and treatment expanded if appropriate.

SUMMARY

Although providers have been using antibiotics for many decades in the setting of PPROM, the optimal regimen remains elusive and will likely continue to evolve. At this time, the recommended regimen includes a 7-day course of ampicillin and erythromycin, with the first 2 days being intravenous and the last 5 being oral. Based on existing data, the substitution of azithromycin does not appear to impact maternal or neonatal outcomes, and has an improved side-effect profile. This regimen is used for PPROM after viability until 34 weeks, for both singletons and multiple gestations. Meta-analyses have shown that antibiotics for this indication are associated with lower rates of maternal and fetal infection, as well as longer pregnancy latency. Thus, latency antibiotics are recommended for all women with PPROM through 34 weeks of gestation.

CLINICS CARE POINTS

- Latency antibiotics are recommended for maternal and fetal benefit when membrane rupture occurs between viability and 34 weeks and 0 days. They can be considered in the setting of previable PPROM with appropriate counseling in the setting of shared decision making.
- Latency antibiotics are not recommended for PPROM after 34 weeks, although GBS prophylaxis remains appropriate.
- The recommended regimen is ampicillin 2 g intravenous every 6 hours × 48 hours, then amoxicillin 250 mg oral every 8 hours × 5 days AND erythromycin 250 mg intravenous every 6 hours × 48 hours, then erythromycin 333 mg oral every 8 hours × 5 days, although many substitute azithromycin.
- In patients with mild PCN allergy, cephalosporins should be used, whereas women with severe allergy can receive 7 days of clindamycin and 2 days of gentamicin as alternatives.

DISCLOSURE

The author has nothing to disclose.

REFERENCES

1. Mercer BM. Preterm premature rupture of the membranes: current approaches to evaluation and management. Obstet Gynecol Clin North Am 2005;32(3):411–28.
2. Kumar D, Moore RM, Mercer BM, et al. The physiology of fetal membrane weakening and rupture: Insights gained from the determination of physical properties revisited. Placenta 2016;42:59–73.
3. Aziz N, Cheng YW, Caughey AB. Neonatal outcomes in the setting of preterm premature rupture of membranes complicated by chorioamnionitis. J Matern Fetal Neonatal Med 2009;22(9):780–4.
4. Reddy UM, Rice MM, Grobman WA, et al. Serious maternal complications after early preterm delivery (24-33 weeks' gestation). Am J Obstet Gynecol 2015; 213(4):538–9.
5. Prelabor rupture of membranes: ACOG practice bulletin, number 217. Obstet Gynecol 2020;135(3):e80–97.
6. Lee J, Romero R, Kim SM, et al. A new antibiotic regimen treats and prevents intra-amniotic inflammation/infection in patients with preterm PROM. J Matern Fetal Neonatal Med 2016;29(17):2727–37.
7. Romero R, Miranda J, Kusanovic JP, et al. Clinical chorioamnionitis at term I: microbiology of the amniotic cavity using cultivation and molecular techniques. J Perinat Med 2015;43(1):19–36.
8. Kim CJ, Romero R, Chaemsaithong P, et al. Acute chorioamnionitis and funisitis: definition, pathologic features, and clinical significance. Am J Obstet Gynecol 2015;213(4 Suppl):S29–52.
9. Sperling RS, Newton E, Gibbs RS. Intraamniotic infection in low-birth-weight infants. J Infect Dis 1988;157(1):113–7.
10. Kenyon S, Boulvain M, Neilson JP. Antibiotics for preterm rupture of membranes. Cochrane Database Syst Rev 2013;(12):CD001058.
11. Kenyon S, Pike K, Jones DR, et al. Childhood outcomes after prescription of antibiotics to pregnant women with preterm rupture of the membranes: 7-year follow-up of the ORACLE I trial. Lancet 2008;372(9646):1310–8.
12. Mercer BM, Miodovnik M, Thurnau GR, et al. Antibiotic therapy for reduction of infant morbidity after preterm premature rupture of the membranes. A randomized controlled trial. National Institute of Child Health and Human Development Maternal-Fetal Medicine Units Network. JAMA 1997;278(12):989–95.
13. Kenyon SL, Taylor DJ, Tarnow-Mordi W, et al. Broad-spectrum antibiotics for preterm, prelabour rupture of fetal membranes: the ORACLE I randomised trial. ORACLE collaborative group. Lancet 2001;357(9261):979–88.
14. Amon E, Lewis SV, Sibai BM, et al. Ampicillin prophylaxis in preterm premature rupture of the membranes: a prospective randomized study. Am J Obstet Gynecol 1988;159(3):539–43.
15. Grable IA, Garcia PM, Perry D, et al. Group B streptococcus and preterm premature rupture of membranes: a randomized, double-blind clinical trial of antepartum ampicillin. Am J Obstet Gynecol 1996;175(4 Pt 1):1036–42.
16. Johnston MM, Sanchez-Ramos L, Vaughn AJ, et al. Antibiotic therapy in preterm premature rupture of membranes: a randomized, prospective, double-blind trial. Am J Obstet Gynecol 1990;163(3):743–7.

17. Ernest JM, Givner LB. A prospective, randomized, placebo-controlled trial of penicillin in preterm premature rupture of membranes. Am J Obstet Gynecol 1994;170(2):516–21.

18. Mercer BM, Moretti ML, Prevost RR, et al. Erythromycin therapy in preterm premature rupture of the membranes: a prospective, randomized trial of 220 patients. Am J Obstet Gynecol 1992;166(3):794–802.

19. Kurki T, Hallman M, Zilliacus R, et al. Premature rupture of the membranes: effect of penicillin prophylaxis and long-term outcome of the children. Am J Perinatol 1992;9(1):11–6.

20. Lockwood CJ, Costigan K, Ghidini A, et al. Double-blind; placebo-controlled trial of piperacillin prophylaxis in preterm membrane rupture. Am J Obstet Gynecol 1993;169(4):970–6.

21. McGregor JA, French JI, Seo K. Antimicrobial therapy in preterm premature rupture of membranes: results of a prospective, double-blind, placebo-controlled trial of erythromycin. Am J Obstet Gynecol 1991;165(3):632–40.

22. Christmas JT, Cox SM, Andrews W, et al. Expectant management of preterm ruptured membranes: effects of antimicrobial therapy. Obstet Gynecol 1992; 80(5):759–62.

23. Lewis DF, Adair CD, Robichaux AG, et al. Antibiotic therapy in preterm premature rupture of membranes: are seven days necessary? a preliminary, randomized clinical trial. Am J Obstet Gynecol 2003;188(6):1413–6 [discussion: 1416–7].

24. Segel SY, Miles AM, Clothier B, et al. Duration of antibiotic therapy after preterm premature rupture of fetal membranes. Am J Obstet Gynecol 2003;189(3): 799–802.

25. Pierson RC, Gordon SS, Haas DM. A retrospective comparison of antibiotic regimens for preterm premature rupture of membranes. Obstet Gynecol 2014; 124(3):515–9.

26. Navathe R, Schoen CN, Heidari P, et al. Azithromycin vs erythromycin for the management of preterm premature rupture of membranes. Am J Obstet Gynecol 2019;221(2):144.e141–8.

27. The obstetrics and gynecology milestone project. J Grad Med Educ 2014;6(1 Supplement 1):129–43.

28. Morris JM, Roberts CL, Bowen JR, et al. Immediate delivery compared with expectant management after preterm pre-labour rupture of the membranes close to term (PPROMT trial): a randomised controlled trial. Lancet 2016;387(10017): 444–52.

29. Quist-Nelson J, de Ruigh AA, Seidler AL, et al. Immediate delivery compared with expectant management in late preterm prelabor rupture of membranes: an individual participant data meta-analysis. Obstet Gynecol 2018;131(2):269–79.

30. Bianco AT, Stone J, Lapinski R, et al. The clinical outcome of preterm premature rupture of membranes in twin versus singleton pregnancies. Am J Perinatol 1996; 13(3):135–8.

31. Mercer BM, Crocker LG, Pierce WF, et al. Clinical characteristics and outcome of twin gestation complicated by preterm premature rupture of the membranes. Am J Obstet Gynecol 1993;168(5):1467–73.

32. Kenyon S, Boulvain M, Neilson J. Antibiotics for preterm premature rupture of membranes. Cochrane Database Syst Rev 2001;(4):CD001058.

33. Myrick O, Dotters-Katz S, Grace M, et al. Prophylactic antibiotics in twin pregnancies complicated by previable preterm premature rupture of membranes. AJP Rep 2016;6(3):e277–82.

34. Obstetric care consensus no. 6 summary: periviable birth. Obstet Gynecol 2017; 130(4):926–8.
35. Dotters-Katz SK, Myrick O, Smid M, et al. Use of prophylactic antibiotics in women with previable prelabor rupture of membranes. J Neonatal Perinatal Med 2017;10(4):431–7.
36. Committee on Practice B-O. ACOG practice bulletin no. 199: use of prophylactic antibiotics in labor and delivery. Obstet Gynecol 2018;132(3):e103–19.
37. Siegel AM, Heine RP, Dotters-Katz SK. The effect of non-penicillin antibiotic regimens on neonatal outcomes in preterm premature rupture of membranes. AJP Rep 2019;9(1):e67–71.
38. Verani JR, McGee L, Schrag SJ, Division of Bacterial Diseases NCfI, Respiratory Diseases CfDC, Prevention. Prevention of perinatal group B streptococcal disease–revised guidelines from CDC, 2010. MMWR Recomm Rep 2010; 59(RR-10):1–36.

Premature Rupture of Membranes with Concurrent Viral Infection

Luke A. Gatta, MD*, Brenna L. Hughes, MD, MSc

KEYWORDS

- Preterm premature rupture of membranes • Hepatitis B virus • Herpes simplex virus
- Human immunodeficiency virus

KEY POINTS

- Treatment of viral infections is geared toward ameliorating maternal symptoms and minimizing perinatal transmission.
- Multidisciplinary teams often are required to manage sequelae due to viral diseases in patients with preterm premature rupture of membranes (PPROM).
- Although data are scarce regarding the antepartum management of common viruses in PPROM, essential principles may be extrapolated from national guidelines and studies in gravid patients. The well-established risks of prematurity are weighed against the often unclear risks of vertical transmission.

INTRODUCTION

Common viral infections have unique considerations during pregnancy. Despite their prevalence, there is a limited understanding of viral mechanisms and the subsequent immunologic response at the maternal-fetal interface. Due to the novel immunity, an otherwise self-limited infection in an adult could confer lifelong morbidity (such as hepatitis B virus) or significant mortality (such as herpes simplex virus [HSV]) in the neonate.

Clinical and bench science data suggest that, under normal circumstances, amniotic fluid is sterile to microorganisms with the use of standard cultivation and molecular microbiologic techniques.[1] In general, viral access into the amnion is presumed by means of 1 of 4 mechanisms: transplacental inoculation by hematogenous spread, introduction through iatrogenic procedures such as amniocentesis, retrograde seeding from the peritoneal cavity via the fallopian tubes, and ascending infection from cervicovaginal secretions.[2] With rupture of membranes (ROM), an ascending infection becomes of particular concern, because the fetus becomes exposed to lower

Funding: This article preparation is unfunded.
Department of Obstetrics and Gynecology, Division of Maternal-Fetal Medicine, Duke University Hospital, 2608 Erwin Road, Durham, NC 27705-4597, USA
* Corresponding author.
E-mail address: luke.gatta@duke.edu

Obstet Gynecol Clin N Am 47 (2020) 605–623
https://doi.org/10.1016/j.ogc.2020.08.006
0889-8545/20/© 2020 Elsevier Inc. All rights reserved.

reproductive tract. Depending on the gestational age at the time of ROM, premature delivery must be weighed against prolonging the pregnancy with expectant management. For this reason, preterm premature ROM (PPROM) with a concurrent maternal viral infection poses a complex risk-benefit situation, which may be summarized as such: the well-established risks of prematurity are weighed against the often unclear risks of vertical transmission. This article reviews several viral infections in pregnancy, with attention to management in the setting of PPROM, with an emphasis on high-quality data and clinical guidelines where available.

HEPATITIS B VIRUS

Hepatitis B virus (HBV) is major global public health concern. In a mortality assessment from 195 countries recently published in *The Lancet*,[3] HBV remains the leading cause of liver disease worldwide. Public health efforts to reduce its global burden focus on perinatal transmission, because the likelihood of developing chronic infection is correlated inversely with age: acutely infected infants without vaccination have an 85% to 95% risk of developing chronic HBV, compared with less than 5% to 15% of otherwise healthy adults.[4] A safe and effective vaccine offers 98% to 100% protection against HBV[4]; therefore, identifying neonates at risk for transmission is of paramount importance.

Natural History and Maternal Impact

HBV is transmitted chiefly through parenteral and sexual contact, because it is present in serum, semen, and saliva. Blood transfusion rarely is implicated.[5] In immunocompetent adults, acute infection generally is mild and self-limited, with symptoms including malaise, anorexia, and nausea. With vague symptoms, evaluation usually is prompted by physical findings, such as jaundice, acholic stools, or darkened urine. Correlated with the onset of symptoms, patients with acute hepatitis may have an increase in liver enzymes (alanine aminotransferase and aspartate aminotransferase) with an increase in serum bilirubin concentration. Mortality of adult patients with acute infection is rare; 85% to 95% of patients have complete resolution, and the remaining 5% to 15% developing chronic infection.[6] With chronic infection, viral replication may continue to manifest in 15% to 30% of patients, leading to cirrhosis.[7]

Screening and Diagnosis

Universal screening for HBV is recommended in pregnancy, assessing hepatitis B surface antigen (HBsAg) during the initial prenatal visit.[8–11] Establishing a diagnosis is more complex and is explained in **Table 1**. The salient points to diagnosis: HBsAg positivity indicates current infection (either acute or chronic), and anti-Hepatitis B surface antibody immunoglobulin G (IgG) confers immunity. HBsAg seropositivity greater than 20 weeks, in the absence of anti-HBs IgG, defines the chronic carrier state.[12] HBV-DNA, a reliable molecular assay of viral replication, is a useful adjunct in assessing disease progression and response to therapy. In pregnancy, HBV-DNA (viral load) is the most important marker for predicting transmission risk.[13,14] In HBsAg-positive women, the Centers for Disease Control and Prevention (CDC), American College of Obstetricians and Gynecologists (ACOG), and Society for Maternal-Fetal Medicine (SMFM) recommend assessing the viral load in the third trimester for consideration of initiating antiviral therapy to decrease vertical transmission.[11,15,16]

Table 1
Establishing hepatitis B diagnosis

	Hepatitis B Surface Antigen	Anti-HBc	Anti-HBs	
Susceptible	Negative	Negative	Negative	
Natural immunity	Negative	Positive	Positive	
Passive immunity	Negative	Negative	Positive	
Acutely infected	Positive	Positive	Negative	Anti-HBc IgM positive
Chronically infected	Positive	Positive	Negative	Anti-HBc IgM negative

Abbreviations: Anti-HBc, Anti-Hepatitis B core antibody; Anti-HBs, Anti-Hepatitis B surface antibody.

Fetal Infection

Vertical transmission includes prenatal, intrapartum, and postpartum mechanisms. The greatest burden of transmission is believed to be the exposure of the neonate to genital tract blood and secretions, without postnatal vaccination.[17–22] Without neonatal prophylaxis, approximately 20% of seropositive women transmit the virus (and approaches 90% if HBeAg is positive).[23] The critical intervention to preventing vertical transmission is a combination of active (HBV vaccine series) and passive (HBV immunoglobulin) immunization in potentially exposed or definitively exposed infants.[11,24]

Treatment in Pregnancy

Similar to nonpregnant counterparts, acute HBV infection in pregnancy typically is mild and self-limited. Treatment mainly is supportive, unless in the setting of severe or protracted liver failure when antiviral therapy may be indicated.[25,26] As demonstrated in the evolution of treatment algorithms for managing viral load in human immunodeficiency virus (HIV), treating chronic HBV increasingly has been focused on reducing viremia, in addition to timely identification of deliveries warranting passive immunoprophylaxis with HBV intravenous immunoglobulin. A meta-analysis of 10 trials demonstrated that a direct-acting antiviral agent (DAA), starting at 24 weeks to 32 weeks, resulted in a decrease in HBV transmission, with an odds ratio (OR) 0.2 (95% CI, 0.10–0.39), when antivirals were combined with immunoprophylaxis. The specific antiviral is beyond the scope of this review, although 4 agents have demonstrated efficacy.[27,28] Current guidelines, from the SMFM and more recently from the American Association for Study of Liver Diseases (AASLD) recommend therapy in highly viremic women (when HBV-DNA threshold is >200,000 IU/mL).[11,29] In all infants born to HBsAg-positive or HBsAg-unknown women, immunoprophylaxis with HBIG and HBV vaccine series should be administered within 12 hours of birth.

Intrapartum Considerations

With an effective and widely used postnatal vaccine, there are scant data regarding labor management strategies to reduce the risk of transmission. Given that the greatest risk of transmission appears to be infected genital tract secretions and blood, it is of theoretic benefit to limit invasive intrapartum procedures. Effective postnatal HBV immunoprophylaxis, however, significantly ameliorates these risks, and the SMFM does not specify a need to alter intrapartum management due to HBsAg positivity.[11]

A 2013 Chinese retrospective study of 1409 infants born to HBsAg-positive mothers with viral load less than 1,000,000 copies/mL did not find a difference in transmission rates with regards to route of delivery.[30,31] There was, however, a significant difference in immunoprophylaxis failure for infants born in highly viremic mothers (>1,000,000 copies/mL) if delivered by elective cesarean (1.4%) compared with vaginal delivery (3.4%) (P = .032). The conclusion of this study must be considered with caution, because the postnatal immunoprophylaxis regimen differs compared with the standard of care in the United States. At this time, given the conflicting data and widespread availability of neonatal immunoprophylaxis, the SMFM does not recommend cesarean delivery for the indication to reduce vertical HBV transmission.[11]

Rupture of Membranes Considerations

The impact of PPROM in vertical transmission of HBV is not well studied, although based on observational data, appears to be negligible. One prospective, observational study of 641 HBsAg-positive women assessed the rate of HBsAg-positive infants at 9 months to 12 months. All women received standard immunoprophylaxis at the time of delivery. Of the 641 cases, 7 infants were HBsAg positive at 9 months to 12 months, each born in the setting of high viremia. When obstetric factors were evaluated, there were no differences between route of delivery or duration of ROM.[32] These findings concur with a retrospective risk analysis of 101 neonates with confirmed vertical transmission, in which ROM was not associated with an increased risk for transmission.[33] Both studies conclude that the length of ROM did not cause a significant effect on the rate of transmission. The most predictive variable appears to be the viral load, and the best therapy remains an antiviral in the setting of high viremia in addition to standard immunoprophylaxis.

Clinical Guidelines

- ACOG, SMFM, and US Preventive Services Task Force (USPSTF) recommend routine prenatal screening by HBsAg.[9–11]
- CDC, ACOG, and SMFM recommend consideration of HBV targeted antiviral therapy in women with a high viral load for the purpose of decreasing the risk of intrauterine fetal infection; grade 2B. AASLD recommends antiviral therapy for mothers with HBV-DNA greater than 200,000 IU/mL.[11,15,34]
- SMFM recommends against cesarean delivery for sole indication to reduce HBV transmission.
- CDC, ACOG, and SMFM recommend universal active immunization of all infants.
- CDC, ACOG, and SMFM recommend HBIG in addition to active immunization to infants born of mothers with known or unknown HBsAg positivity.

HEPATITIS C VIRUS

Hepatitis C virus (HCV) is the most common blood-borne infection in the United States[35] and the leading cause of chronic liver disease. Its increasing prevalence is linked to the opioid epidemic.[36] Although no effective vaccine exists, the development of DAAs within the past decade have expanded treatment options with improved cure rates and morbidity from both the disease as well as treatment. The role of treatment during pregnancy remains an active area of research.

Natural History and Maternal Impact

HCV transmission is primarily by percutaneous exposure, most commonly through sharing contaminated needles. It is transmitted less efficiently through sexual intercourse and transmitted rarely with blood transfusion. Acute infection largely is asymptomatic, although 25% of cases present with vague symptoms, including abdominal pain, anorexia, or malaise.[9] The first 6 months after exposure to HCV is considered an acute infection, with approximately 15% to 45% of acutely infected individuals spontaneously clearing the virus within 6 months.[37] The remaining develop chronic HCV, which, although typically asymptomatic, may progress to cirrhosis within 20 years in 15% to 30% of individuals.[38] Likely due to immune changes, pregnancy is associated with a delayed progression to fibrosis.[39–41]

Screening and Diagnosis

After exposure, anti-HCV antibodies develop within 2 months to 6 months and persist indefinitely. Positive serology may indicate active HCV infection, chronic HCV infection, or natural immunity[42] and should be reflexively followed by an assessment for viremia using quantitative HCV-RNA. Additionally, HCV genotyping should also be performed to guide resistance patterns and treatment decisions.

The ideal screening strategy in pregnancy is controversial. Ideally, due to the absence of available treatment during pregnancy, women with HCV would be identified and treatment initiated prior to conception.[9,43] In a recent Maternal-Fetal Medicine Units study of HCV mother-to-child transmission, including 106,842 women, the antibody seroprevalence rate was 2.4 cases per 1000 women,[44] and the most sensitive risk factors for HCV positivity included injection drug use (adjusted OR [aOR] 22.9; 95% CI, 8.2 to 64.0), blood transfusion (aOR 3.7; 95% CI, 1.3–10.4), tobacco use (aOR 2.4; 95% CI, 1.2–4.6), partner with HCV (aOR 6.3, 95% CI 1.8–22.6), and more than 3 lifetime prior sexual partners (aOR 5.3 [95% CI 1.4–19.8]). A recent meta-analysis noted, however, that 27% of women may have no identifiable risk factors; therefore, the role of universal screening currently is under debate.[45] At present, the Infectious Diseases Society of America (IDSA) recommends universal testing, ideally at the prenatal visit.[46] This year, the USPSTF and CDC updated their recommendations to include universal screening in pregnant patients greater than 18 years[47] in areas where the HCV prevalence is greater than 0.1%,[48] although the USPSTF recommends 1-time screening whereas the CDC recommends screening with each pregnancy. Although the screening strategy is controversial, it is clear that, in the present absence of available treatment of pregnant woman, a diagnosis of HCV does not necessarily translate into a cure or reduction in perinatal transmission.

Fetal Infection

Vertical transmission of HCV is assumed to be a risk for women with viremia. One meta-analysis of 25 studies found a risk of transmission in women with detectable HCV-RNA to be 5.8% (95% CI, 4.2, 7.8).[49] In those studies, only 1 neonate (out of a cohort of 473, or 0.21%) was diagnosed with vertically acquired HCV infection when the mother had negative HCV-RNA, and this was felt to be due to laboratory error in measuring maternal viral load. Several studies demonstrate that a higher quantitative HCV-RNA is correlated with a higher risk of transmission.[50,51] Concurrent HIV infection is a known cofactor for vertical transmission, with OR 1.97 to 2.82 compared with non–HIV-infected counterparts.[52] There is no effective immunoglobulin or vaccine available.

Treatment in Pregnancy

The standard of care for the treatment of chronic HCV changed in 2011 with the advent of DAAs. Prior to this, pegylated interferon and ribavirin were used, which achieved a sustained virologic response (or undetectable HCV-RNA) in 40% to 80% of treated patients.[53] With DAAs, HCV was declared to be a curable disease, with greater than 90% sustained virologic response observed, depending on the HCV genotype and disease severity.[54] Furthermore, fewer side effects than interferon-based modalities were observed. The specific DAA and generation used are beyond the scope of this review.

DAAs are not yet approved for use in pregnancy, and regimens used are reserved in the setting of clinical trials. If a woman becomes pregnant while undergoing treatment with DAA, however, she may continue with appropriate counseling. Although animal studies do not suggest teratogenic risk, human data are limited.[55] In the first phase I study released this year evaluating DAA treatment during pregnancy, no adverse outcomes were identified in the 9 patients initiating DAA therapy at 23 weeks' to 24 weeks' gestation.[56] If a woman is identified to be HCV positive during pregnancy, treatment typically is deferred to the postpartum period. Ribavirin is contraindicated in pregnancy due to teratogenic effects demonstrated in animal species.[57]

Intrapartum Considerations

The mode of delivery—cesarean versus vaginal—has not been shown to be a risk factor for vertical transmission of HCV[58]; therefore, cesarean delivery to reduce HCV transmission is not recommended.[43] Interventions in labor management may be associated, however, with an increased risk of transmission. One retrospective study[59] reported that internal fetal monitoring was associated with increased risk of transmission compared with no internal monitoring. A separate retrospective study, however, found no association.[60] Based on the available evidence and without available postnatal prophylaxis, the risks generally outweigh the benefits at term and the SMFM recommends that obstetric care providers avoid internal fetal monitoring and episiotomy in managing labor in HCV-positive women when feasible.[43]

Rupture of Membranes Considerations

Data on risk of ROM on vertical transmission are conflicting. One prospective study of 9 infants born to HCV-positive mothers reported that membrane rupture for greater than 6 hours was associated with increased risk of vertical transmission (OR 9.3; 95% CI, 1.5 to 179.7).[61] Another study of 6 HCV-infected infants also found an association between duration of ruptured membranes and transmission, with median 18 hours from the time of rupture to delivery.[62] In contrast to these 2 studies, another retrospective study of risks of perinatal transmission in 17 HCV-infected infants did not see a difference with ROM greater than 6 hours.[59] These data agreed with a prospective study of 212 HCV-infected mothers, with 12 infected neonates in the cohort.[63] In this study, viral load and HIV were identified as independent risk factors, and the duration of ROM did not confer additional risk. In conclusion, based on potential risks, the SMFM states that patients with ROM at term should not be expectantly managed, although acknowledging that data are inadequate in the setting of PPROM. Given the low rate of transmission and conflicting data in the literature, however, both the ACOG and SMFM state that usual obstetric management should not be altered in the setting of PPROM (Table 2).[43]

Clinical Guidelines

- CDC, USPSTF, and IDSA recommend universal screening in pregnancy by testing anti-HCV antibodies.
- SMFM recommends that DAAs be used in the setting of a clinical trial, and initiation be deferred to the postpartum period until further data demonstrate safety
- SMFM recommends that obstetric care providers avoid internal fetal monitoring, episiotomy, or early amniotomy (at term).
- SMFM and ACOG recommend against cesarean delivery solely for the indication of HCV.

Table 2
Key points in management of common viral infections

	Hepatitis B Virus	Hepatitis C Virus	Human Immunodeficiency Virus	Herpes Simplex Virus
Antepartum therapy	• Repeat viral load in third trimester. • Consider therapy when HBV-DNA threshold >200,000 IU/mL.	• Therapy is not yet approved for use in pregnancy (only phase I data available to date). • Initiate DAA in postpartum • Can continue DAA treatment if started prior to pregnancy	• Initiate ART as soon as diagnosis is established.	• Initiate oral suppression at 36 wk to reduce the risk of shedding.
Intrapartum management	• With appropriate postnatal immunoprophylaxis, no changes to intrapartum management • Cesarean delivery per routine obstetric management	• Risks of internal monitoring, episiotomy generally outweigh benefits. • Cesarean delivery per routine obstetric management	If viral load <1000 copies/mL • No changes to intrapartum management • Consider ZDV prophylaxis. If viral load >1000 copies/mL • Recommend prelabor cesarean delivery • Recommend ZDV prophylaxis. • Risks of internal monitoring, episiotomy generally outweigh benefits	• With prodromal symptoms, active lesions, recommend cesarean delivery. • If primary outbreak occurs in the third trimester, consider cesarean delivery.

HUMAN IMMUNODEFICIENCY VIRUS

Antiretroviral therapy (ART) has changed the landscape for management of HIV-positive patients dramatically, including during pregnancy. Fortified by longitudinal data, ART and multidisciplinary delivery planning have been demonstrated to both improve maternal outcomes and decrease the perinatal transmission rate. Academic resources are widely available to clinicians. Among these are the National Institutes of Health perinatal guidelines[64] and the National Clinician Consultation Center, which operates a 24/7 perinatal HIV consultation hotline (888-448-8765) to assist with complex and time-sensitive medical decision-making[65] on labor and delivery units.

Natural History and Maternal Impact

HIV usually is acquired through percutaneous exposure, sexual intercourse, or perinatal transmission. Up to 60% of acute infections are asymptomatic, with the remaining having a mononucleosis-like illness characterized by fever, myalgia, and headache. During the initial infection, HIV rapidly infects CD4 cells, leading to a transient drop. After early infection and seroconversion, there is a period of chronic HIV infection that is characterized by a progressive waning of CD4 count as the virus subclinically replicates. In the absence of ART, the time from inoculation to the development of severe immunosuppression when CD4 count less than 200 cells/cubic millimeter is approximately 8 years to 10 years.[66] There does not appear to be an impact of pregnancy on the natural history of HIV, because prospective data in pregnant and matched nonpregnant controls were similar with regards to patient symptoms and laboratory values, including CD4 and viral load.[67]

Screening and Diagnosis

The ACOG recommends routine testing for HIV, using an opt-out approach with an antibody-antigen combination screening test,[68-70] with a repeat test ordered in the third trimester in patients at risk or residing in high-incidence areas. Furthermore, the CDC recommends rapid (within 1-hour) screening if a woman present to labor with unknown HIV status.[69] If results are positive and confirmed, follow-up laboratory tests should include $CD4^+$, viral load, and resistance testing as well as testing for alternative sexually transmitted infections.[70]

In patients known to be positive, HIV-RNA levels should be monitored throughout pregnancy. If HIV-RNA viral loads are detectable, viral load should be repeated monthly until negative. If HIV-RNA levels are undetectable, viral load should be repeated every 3 months throughout pregnancy. In all subjects, HIV-RNA levels should be assessed at approximately 34 weeks' to 36 weeks' gestation to guide delivery planning.[64]

Fetal Transmission

Without treatment, the perinatal transmission rate has been demonstrated to be 25%.[71] Although the precise mechanisms of perinatal transmission are unknown, research suggests that intrapartum exposure leads to a disproportionate burden of transmission compared with congenital or postnatal infection, and data indicate that the rate of perinatal transmission is correlated to the RNA viremia.[72] Microtransfusion of blood during uterine contraction or cervicovaginal secretions have been proposed.[73]

Treatment in Pregnancy

In the era of ART, the care of women with HIV has demonstrated favorable maternal outcomes and historically low rates of vertical transmission. Many women enter pregnancy aware of their status and already sustained on an effective ART regimen. For treatment-naive women, it is recommended to begin ART as soon as possible after diagnosis.[74–76] Specific regimens are beyond the scope of this review and depend on viral resistance profile, interactions with other medications, and socioeconomic factors. Certain regimens are preferred in pregnancy given longitudinal pharmacokinetic data, which are updated by the Department of Health and Human Services.[64]

Intrapartum Consideration

Intrapartum management is dependent on viral load. Based on observational data, a viral load threshold (<1000 copies/mL) has been shown to minimize vertical transmission,[77,78] with data suggesting a less than 1% risk of perinatal transmission.[75] There is no change to delivery planning, and women may await spontaneous labor or undergo an induction of labor without conferring additional risk of transmission.[79]

Management bifurcates, however, in women with viral loads greater than 1000 copies/mL. In these patients, perinatal transmission may be reduced by performing a prelabor cesarean delivery. Quality data, including 1 randomized controlled trial (RCT)[80] and 1 meta-analysis,[81] note that a scheduled, prelabor cesarean delivery reduced the risk of transmission. The ACOG recommends a delivery at 38 weeks' gestation, intentionally to avoid labor.[82] Once advanced labor or prolonged ROM has occurred, the benefit of cesarean for preventing transmission is lost.[72] Furthermore, patients with an elevated viral load should be treated with intrapartum zidovudine (ZDV). The landmark Pediatric AIDS Clinical Trials Group Protocol 076[71] found that the use of ZDV reduces the transmission rate from 25% in placebo cohort, to 8% in the treatment group.

Although ZDV is not required for HIV-positive women with suppressed viral loads, certain academic centers may elect to make this routine practice. The ACOG committee opinion opines that the intrapartum administration of ZDV to patients with a low (<1000 copies/mL) or suppressed viral load is dependent on expert opinion and clinical judgment.[82]

As with other viral infections, obstetric procedures, including internal monitoring or episiotomy, have been suggested to increase the risk for vertical transmission. Regardless of viral suppression, the ACOG recommends avoiding their use.

Rupture of Membranes Considerations

Observational data prior to the routine use of ART found an association between the duration of ROM and the risk of transmission.[83–85] In the era of ART, however, this risk was ameliorated. One prospective[86] study in 210 women with a suppressed viral load (<1000 copies/mL) did not demonstrate transmission in women with prolonged ROM, regardless of the mode of delivery. It, therefore, is extrapolated that the role of suppression outweighs the risk from ruptured membranes. This also applies to preterm rupture. In a study of 260 preterm deliveries in HIV-positive women, there were no cases of perinatal transmission[87] in the setting of undetectable viral load, despite the longer duration of ROM (the median [interquartile range] duration of ROM in the cohort rupturing before 34 weeks was 16 [2–55] hours).

Management of ruptured membranes in women with viral loads greater than greater than 1000 copies/mL is more challenging. Although scheduled cesarean delivery rates have been demonstrated to reduce transmission, data are unclear whether there is benefit of cesarean delivery after ROM. In a study of the mode of delivery among 5131 deliveries not stratified by viral load, the rate of transmission in elective cesarean deliveries was 0.8%, compared with 1.6% for urgent cesarean deliveries and 1.9% for vaginal deliveries.[88] In 1 retrospective study of 18 subjects with HIV who had PPROM prior to 34 weeks' gestation, duration of ruptured membranes was not demonstrated to be a predictor: in the 2 cases of perinatal transmission, 1 occurred after 24 hours ROM, and the other was 2 weeks. In both cases, the viral load was greater than 1000 copies/mL and delivery was performed by cesarean. Because data are not clear whether cesarean delivery after labor or ruptured membranes reduces transmission, care is individualized and should be made via a shared decision-making process with the patient (**Table 3**).[65]

Clinical Guidelines

- ACOG, CDC, and USPSTF recommend universal screening, with repeat screening in third trimester for women with risk factors or living in high-incidence areas.
- ACOG recommends that HIV-RNA levels in pregnant women should be monitored at the initial prenatal visit, 2 weeks to 4 weeks after initiating (or changing) combination ART drug regimens; monthly until RNA levels are undetectable; and then at least every 3 months during pregnancy.
- ACOG recommends shared decision-making for delivery: if viral loads less than 1000 copies/mL, mode of delivery or ROM are not predictive of transmission. If viral load greater than 1000 copies/mL, women should be offered a prelabor cesarean delivery at 38 0/7 weeks, and receive ZDV prophylaxis.
- Rapid screening (within 1 hour) should be available at labor and delivery units.

HERPES SIMPLEX VIRUS

Genital HSV generally poses a low maternal risk and is a concern primarily to the newborn because it may cause serious morbidity and mortality. In adults, HSV is a common, lifelong, and often asymptomatic infection. Traditionally, HSV-1 was attributed to be the cause of orolabial lesions, and HSV-2 was thought to be the etiology of genital lesions and associated with birth-related risks. Genital infections due to HSV-1 are increasing,[89] however, and for the purposes of this review, HSV assumes either HSV-1 or HSV-2 infection.

Natural History and Transmission

Genital HSV is transmitted almost exclusively through sexual contact from mucosa of abraded skin, replicating within the epidermis. With primary infection, the virus inoculates the sensory ganglia, becoming a latent infection. Reactivation may occur throughout the lifetime, manifesting as painful ulcerative lesions. Because only 20% to 30% of patients may have symptoms,[90] the true incidence of HSV is difficult to determine, although 2015 to 2016 National Health and Nutrition Examination Survey estimates that 48.1% and 12.1% of Americans have HSV-1 and HSV-2, respectively. Women are more likely than men to have HSV-2, owing to the more efficient transmission from male to female.[91] The natural history often includes frequent recurrences, although there is substantial variability among patients. In women with prior history of HSV, 75% may expect an episode of recurrence during the pregnancy without treatment.[92]

Screening and Diagnosis

Routine serologic or laboratory testing is not recommended in pregnancy, owing to the high incidence, the lack of cure, and the widespread availability of generic oral antivirals to treat recurrent symptoms. It is recommended that, during prenatal care, all women are screened about a history of HSV symptoms.[93]

Table 3
Considerations with rupture of membranes

	Hepatitis B Virus	Hepatitis C Virus	Human Immunodeficiency Virus	Herpes Simplex Virus
ROM at term (≥37 wk)	Do not delay delivery.	Do not delay delivery.	Do not delay delivery.	Do not delay delivery.
ROM, late preterm (≥34 wk)	Do not delay delivery.	Do not delay delivery.	Do not delay delivery.	Do not delay delivery.
ROM, preterm (<34 wk)	• No indication for expedited delivery by HBsAg alone • In a patient with high viremia, consider antiviral therapy.	• No indication for expedited delivery by HCV alone	• No indication for expedited delivery by HIV alone • Emphasis on viral load suppression with ART • In women with viral load >1000 copies mL, because data are not clear whether cesarean delivery after ROM reduces transmission, care is individualized. Optimizing ART regimen and adherence are prioritized.	• No indication for expedited delivery by HSV alone • In a patient without active lesions, manage per normal indications. Initiate suppressive therapy. • In a patient with active lesions, start treatment doses. Low threshold to move forward with cesarean delivery with the onset of labor

When a patient presents with clinical symptoms, type-specific serologic and direct virologic assays are required in order to establish a diagnosis. In the setting of an active genital ulcer, the vesicle may be unroofed and swabbed sent for polymerase chain reaction (PCR) testing, which has improved sensitivity compared with viral culture.[94,95] If the swab results are positive for HSV, but the HSV-1 and HSV-2 antibodies are negative, the patient has a primary infection. If HSV is recovered from the genital lesion, and there are preexisting antibodies in the serum, the infection is considered to be recurrent. Classifying the infection as primary or recurrent is important, because the former has a higher risk for neonatal transmission, with OR 33.1 (95% CI, 6.5–168) in a study of 202 women with HSV at the time of labor.[96] Women with a history of laboratory-confirmed HSV do not warrant testing in the setting of highly suspicious lesion.

Fetal and Neonatal Transmission

Perinatal transmission occurs with direct contact from infected sites. The highest risk of infection is conferred in the setting of primary outbreak at the time of delivery, ranging from 30% to 60%.[97] The transmission risk is reduced significantly in the setting of recurrent infection, ranging from 1.3% to 3%, likely due to a mitigating effect from HSV-specific antibodies and a lower concentration of the virus.[98,99] For women with a history of HSV but no visible lesion at delivery, the transmission risk has been estimated to be 2/10,000.[100] Congenital infections rarely have been reported, and in 1 of the largest case series of 36 neonates with congenital herpes, ultrasound findings are nonspecific.[101,102]

Treatment in Pregnancy

Although an outbreak generally is self-limited, treatment with antiviral therapy can reduce the severity and duration of the symptoms, particularly with primary infection. Empiric treatment generally is recommended in the setting of primary disease while awaiting virologic testing.[93] For recurrent disease in the first and second trimesters, because the outbreak generally is self-limited, patients may opt to defer treatment as to reduce exposure to medication, although patient symptoms always are an indication for treatment.

In all women with a history of HSV outbreak during pregnancy, suppressive therapy is indicated to reduce viral shedding, recurrent outbreak, and the need for cesarean delivery.[92] A Cochrane meta-analysis of 7 RCTs comparing suppressive treatment to placebo demonstrated a reduced risk of clinical recurrence (RR 0.28; 95% CI, 0.18–0.43) and cesarean delivery (RR 0.30; 95% CI, 0.20–0.45),[92] although there was no effect seen on neonatal HSV likely due to the low disease prevalence.

Intrapartum Considerations

In the setting of prodromal symptoms or in the presence of active lesions, both the ACOG and CDC recommend cesarean delivery.[103,104] Because the presence of viral shedding has been demonstrated to confer intrapartum transmission, women with a history of HSV should be asked about prodromal symptoms and subsequently examined in order to detect active lesions at the time of admission to labor and delivery. One RCT has demonstrated that the route of delivery has a significant impact on the rate of transmission.[96] In 202 women with active HSV outbreak at the time of delivery, cesarean delivery was associated with a lower rate of transmission 1/85 (1.2%) compared with vaginal delivery 9/117 (7.7%) (P = .047). In women with a history of HSV but without active lesions or prodromal symptoms, cesarean delivery is not indicated. The most recent ACOG practice bulletin, updated May 2020, noted that women with a primary or first-episode genital HSV during the third trimester may be offered cesarean due to the possibility of prolonged viral shedding.[104] A PCR test for viral shedding prior to planned delivery also could be considered.

Rupture of Membranes

In a patient without active lesions on examination or prodromal symptoms, ROM may be managed per normal obstetric indications, including during the preterm setting. In women with active lesions, although data demonstrate that cesarean delivery reduces the risk of transmission by approximately 75%, there are no data on neonatal outcomes when cesarean delivery is completed in the setting of labor or ruptured membranes.[105] When at term, cesarean delivery should ensue as soon as feasible after ROM.[104]

One observational study followed 29 subjects with recurrent herpetic lesions who developed PPROM at median 28.7 weeks (range, 24.6–31.0), with a median latency period of 13.2 (range, 1–35) days from outbreak to delivery.[106] Cesarean delivery was completed in 13 (45%) cases due to persistent HSV lesions and 16 (55%) had vaginal delivery after resolution in symptoms. In this cohort, there were no cases of neonatal herpes and the neonatal HSV cultures were all negative. Neonatal morbidity was, as expected, attributed to prematurity. A total of 8 patients in this study were treated with acyclovir in this cohort, due to patient symptoms. The recent ACOG practice bulletin recommends (level C evidence) suppressive treatment when expectant management is pursued, starting as soon as possible after ROM is confirmed.

CLINICAL GUIDELINES

- ACOG recommends type-specific testing of suspicious lesions; in patients with a history of HSV, testing is not indicated.
- ACOG and CDC recommend that women with HSV be offered suppressive therapy at 36 gestation, or after primary outbreak if it occurs in the third trimester.
- ACOG recommends cesarean delivery in the setting of active genital lesions or prodromal symptoms. Cesarean delivery is not recommended in women without active lesions. For women with a primary outbreak in the third trimester (but without present symptoms), cesarean delivery may be considered.
- In women expectantly managed with ruptured membranes, treatment with an antiviral is recommended as soon as ROM is confirmed.

DISCLOSURE

The authors have nothing to disclose.

CLINICS CARE POINTS

- For viral infections in the setting of PPROM, the well-established risks of prematurity are weighed against the often unclear risks of vertical transmission.
- The risk of vertical transmission of viral infections do not indicate expedited delivery in the setting of PPROM before 34 weeks gestation. Efforts may be aimed at reducing maternal viremia.
- Recommendations regarding the mode of delivery depend on the virus itself. For example, cesarean delivery is not recommended for the sole indication of Hepatitis B Virus and Hepatitis C Virus, but may be recommended in HIV in the setting of an elevated viral load.

REFERENCES

1. Kim CJ, Romero R, Chaemsaithong P, et al. Acute chorioamnionitis and funisitis: definition, pathologic features, and clinical significance. Am J Obstet Gynecol 2015;213(4 Suppl):S29–52.
2. Racicot K, Mor G. Risks associated with viral infections during pregnancy. J Clin Invest 2017;127(5):1591–9.
3. GBD 2017 Cirrhosis Collaborators. The global, regional, and national burden of cirrhosis by cause in 195 countries and territories, 1990-2017: a systematic analysis for the Global Burden of Disease Study 2017. Lancet Gastroenterol Hepatol 2020;5(3):245–66.
4. World Health Organization. Hepatitis B. 2019. Available at: https://www.who.int/news-room/fact-sheets/detail/hepatitis-b. Accessed April 9, 2020.
5. Schreiber GB, Busch MP, Kleinman SH, et al. The risk of transfusion-transmitted viral infections. The Retrovirus Epidemiology Donor Study. N Engl J Med 1996; 334(26):1685–90.
6. Sookoian S. Liver disease during pregnancy: acute viral hepatitis. Ann Hepatol 2006;5(3):231–6.
7. Keeffe EB, Dieterich DT, Han SH, et al. A treatment algorithm for the management of chronic hepatitis B virus infection in the United States: 2008 update. Clin Gastroenterol Hepatol 2008;6(12):1315–41.
8. Mast EE, Weinbaum CM, Fiore AE, et al. A comprehensive immunization strategy to eliminate transmission of hepatitis B virus infection in the United States: recommendations of the Advisory Committee on Immunization Practices (ACIP) Part II: immunization of adults. MMWR Recomm Rep 2006;55(RR-16):1–33 [quiz: CE1–4].
9. ACOG Practice Bulletin No 86. Viral hepatitis in pregnancy. Obstet Gynecol 2007;110(4):941–56.
10. Lin K, Vickery J. Screening for hepatitis B virus infection in pregnant women: evidence for the U.S. Preventive Services Task Force reaffirmation recommendation statement. Ann Intern Med 2009;150(12):874–6.
11. Society for Maternal Fetal Medicine Consult Series No 38: Hepatitis B in pregnancy screening, treatment, and prevention of vertical transmission. Am J Obstet Gynecol 2016;214(1):6–14.
12. Center for Disease Control. Sexually transmitted diseases treatment guidelines, 2006. MMWR Recomm Rep 2006;55(RR-11):1–94.
13. Wiseman E, Fraser MA, Holden S, et al. Perinatal transmission of hepatitis B virus: an Australian experience. Med J Aust 2009;190(9):489–92.
14. Patel NH, Joshi SS, Lau KC, et al. Analysis of serum hepatitis B virus RNA levels in a multiethnic cohort of pregnant chronic hepatitis B carriers. J Clin Virol 2019; 111:42–7.
15. Schillie S, Vellozzi C, Reingold A, et al. Prevention of Hepatitis B Virus Infection in the United States: Recommendations of the Advisory Committee on Immunization Practices. MMWR Recomm Rep 2017;67.
16. ACOG Practice Advisory. Hepatitis B Prevention. 2018. Available at: https://www.acog.org/clinical/clinical-guidance/practice   advisory/articles/2018/01/hepatitis-b-prevention. Accessed June 14, 2020.
17. Lin HH, Lee TY, Chen DS, et al. Transplacental leakage of HBeAg-positive maternal blood as the most likely route in causing intrauterine infection with hepatitis B virus. J Pediatr 1987;111(6 Pt 1):877–81.

18. Xu DZ, Yan YP, Choi BC, et al. Risk factors and mechanism of transplacental transmission of hepatitis B virus: a case-control study. J Med Virol 2002; 67(1):20–6.

19. Bhat P, Anderson DA. Hepatitis B virus translocates across a trophoblastic barrier. J Virol 2007;81(13):7200–7.

20. Cheung KW, Seto MT, Wong SF. Towards complete eradication of hepatitis B infection from perinatal transmission: review of the mechanisms of in utero infection and the use of antiviral treatment during pregnancy. Eur J Obstet Gynecol Reprod Biol 2013;169(1):17–23.

21. Shao Q, Zhao X, Li M D. Role of peripheral blood mononuclear cell transportation from mother to baby in HBV intrauterine infection. Arch Gynecol Obstet 2013;288(6):1257–61.

22. Wong F, Pai R, Schalkwyk K, et al. Hepatitis B in pregnancy: a concise review of neonatal vertical transmission and antiviral prophylaxis. Ann Hepatol 2014; 13(2):187–95.

23. Jonas MM. Hepatitis B and pregnancy: an underestimated issue. Liver Int 2009; 29(Suppl 1):133–9.

24. Beasley RP, Hwang LY, Stevens CE, et al. Efficacy of hepatitis B immune globulin for prevention of perinatal transmission of the hepatitis B virus carrier state: final report of a randomized double-blind, placebo-controlled trial. Hepatology 1983;3(2):135–41.

25. Degertekin B, Lok AS. Indications for therapy in hepatitis B. Hepatology 2009; 49(5 Suppl):S129–37.

26. Brady CW. Liver Disease in Pregnancy: What's New. Hepatol Commun 2020; 4(2):145–56.

27. Ayres A, Yuen L, Jackson KM, et al. Short duration of lamivudine for the prevention of hepatitis B virus transmission in pregnancy: lack of potency and selection of resistance mutations. J Viral Hepat 2014;21(11):809–17.

28. Potthoff A, Rifai K, Wedemeyer H, et al. Successful treatment of fulminant hepatitis B during pregnancy. Z Gastroenterol 2009;47(7):667–70.

29. Terrault NA, Lok ASF, McMahon BJ, et al. Update on prevention, diagnosis, and treatment of chronic hepatitis B: AASLD 2018 hepatitis B guidance. Hepatology 2018;67(4):1560–99.

30. Pan CQ, Zou HB, Chen Y, et al. Cesarean section reduces perinatal transmission of hepatitis B virus infection from hepatitis B surface antigen-positive women to their infants. Clin Gastroenterol Hepatol 2013;11(10):1349–55.

31. Yang J, Zeng M, Men Y, et al. Elective caesarean section versus vaginal delivery for preventing mother to child transmission of hepatitis B virus–a systematic review. Virol J 2008;5:100.

32. Cheung KW, Seto MTY, So PL, et al. The effect of rupture of membranes and labour on the risk of hepatitis B vertical transmission: Prospective multicentre observational study. Eur J Obstet Gynecol Reprod Biol 2019;232:97–100.

33. Guo Z, Shi XH, Feng YL, et al. Risk factors of HBV intrauterine transmission among HBsAg-positive pregnant women. J Viral Hepat 2013;20(5):317–21.

34. ACOG Practice Advisory. Hepatits B Prevention. 2018. Available at: https://www.acog.org/clinical/clinical-guidance/practice-advisory/articles/2018/01/hepatitis-b-prevention. Accessed June 15, 2020.

35. Hofmeister MG, Rosenthal EM, Barker LK, et al. Estimating Prevalence of Hepatitis C Virus Infection in the United States, 2013-2016. Hepatology 2019;69(3): 1020–31.

36. Zibbell JE, Asher AK, Patel RC, et al. Increases in Acute Hepatitis C Virus Infection Related to a Growing Opioid Epidemic and Associated Injection Drug Use, United States, 2004 to 2014. Am J Public Health 2018;108(2):175–81.

37. World Health Organization. Guidelines for the screening, care and treatment of persons with hepatitis C infection. Geneva (Switzerland): World Health Organization; 2014.

38. van der Meer AJ, Veldt BJ, Feld JJ, et al. Association between sustained virological response and all-cause mortality among patients with chronic hepatitis C and advanced hepatic fibrosis. JAMA 2012;308(24):2584–93.

39. Resti M, Azzari C, Mannelli F, et al. Mother to child transmission of hepatitis C virus: prospective study of risk factors and timing of infection in children born to women seronegative for HIV-1. Tuscany Study Group on Hepatitis C Virus Infection. BMJ 1998;317(7156):437–41.

40. Sangiovanni G, Prati GM, Fasani P, et al. The natural history of compensated cirrhosis due to hepatitis C virus: A 17-year cohort study of 214 patients. Hepatology 2006;43(6):1303–10.

41. Gervais A, Bacq Y, Bernau J, et al. Decrease in serum ALT and increase in serum HCV RNA during pregnancy in women with chronic hepatitis C. J Hepatol 2000;32(2):293–9.

42. Center for Disease Control. Testing for HCV infection: an update of guidance for clinicians and laboratorians. MMWR Morb Mortal Wkly Rep 2013;62(18):362–5.

43. Society for Maternal Fetal Medicine Consult Series No 42. Hepatitis C in pregnancy: screening, treatment, and management. Am J Obstet Gynecol 2017; 217(5):B2–12.

44. Prasad M, Saade GR, Sandoval G, et al. Hepatitis C Virus Antibody Screening in a Cohort of Pregnant Women: Identifying Seroprevalence and Risk Factors. Obstet Gynecol 2020;135(4):778–88.

45. Andes A, Ellenberg K, Vakos A, et al. Hepatitis C Virus in Pregnancy: A Systematic Review of the Literature. Am J Perinatol 2020.

46. AASLD-IDSA Hepatitis C Guidance Panel. Hepatitis C Guidance 2018 Update: AASLD-IDSA Recommendations for Testing, Managing, and Treating Hepatitis C Virus Infection. Clin Infect Dis 2018;67(10):1477–92.

47. Chou R, Dana T, Fu R, et al. Screening for Hepatitis C Virus Infection in Adolescents and Adults: Updated Evidence Report and Systematic Review for the US Preventive Services Task Force. JAMA 2020;323(10):976–91.

48. Schillie S, Wester C, Osborne M, et al. CDC Recommendations for Hepatitis C Screening Among Adults - United States, 2020. MMWR Recomm Rep 2020; 69(2):1–17.

49. BEnova L, Mohamoud YA, Calvert C, et al. Vertical transmission of hepatitis C virus: systematic review and meta-analysis. Clin Infect Dis 2014;59(6):765–73.

50. Ohto H, Terazawa S, Sasaki N, et al. Transmission of hepatitis C virus from mothers to infants. The Vertical Transmission of Hepatitis C Virus Collaborative Study Group. N Engl J Med 1994;330(11):744–50.

51. Yeung ST, King SM, Roberts EA. Mother-to-infant transmission of hepatitis C virus. Hepatology 2001;34(2):223–9.

52. Pappalardo BL. Influence of maternal human immunodeficiency virus (HIV) co-infection on vertical transmission of hepatitis C virus (HCV): a meta-analysis. Int J Epidemiol 2003;32(5):727–34.

53. European Association for Study of the Liver. Recommendations on Treatment of Hepatitis C. J Hepatol 2015;63(1):199–236.

54. Li DK, Chung RT. Overview of Direct-Acting Antiviral Drugs and Drug Resistance of Hepatitis C Virus. Methods Mol Biol 2019;1911:3–32.
55. Spera AM, Eldin TK, Tosone G, et al. Antiviral therapy for hepatitis C: Has anything changed for pregnant/lactating women? World J Hepatol 2016;8(12): 557–65.
56. ClinicalTrials.gov. Study of hepatitis C treatment during pregnancy (HIP) 2020. Available at: https://www.clinicaltrials.gov/ct2/show/NCT02683005. Accessed May 1, 2020.
57. Sinclair SM, Jones JK, Miller RK, et al. The Ribavirin Pregnancy Registry: An Interim Analysis of Potential Teratogenicity at the Mid-Point of Enrollment. Drug Saf 2017;40(12):1205–18.
58. Cottrell EB, Chou R, Wasson N, et al. Reducing risk for mother-to-infant transmission of hepatitis C virus: a systematic review for the U.S. Preventive Services Task Force. Ann Intern Med 2013;158(2):109–13.
59. Garcia-Tejedor A, Maiques-Montesinos V, Diago-Amela VJ, et al. Risk factors for vertical transmission of hepatitis C virus: a single center experience with 710 HCV-infected mothers. Eur J Obstet Gynecol Reprod Biol 2015;194:173–7.
60. Foster GR, Tudor-Williams G, White J, et al. Effects of mode of delivery and infant feeding on the risk of mother-to-child transmission of hepatitis C virus. BJOG 2003;110(1):91 [author reply 91].
61. Mast EE, Hwang LY, Seto DS, et al. Risk factors for perinatal transmission of hepatitis C virus (HCV) and the natural history of HCV infection acquired in infancy. J Infect Dis 2005;192(11):1880–9.
62. Spencer JD, Latt N, Beeby PJ, et al. Transmission of hepatitis C virus to infants of human immunodeficiency virus-negative intravenous drug-using mothers: rate of infection and assessment of risk factors for transmission. J Viral Hepat 1997;4(6):395–409.
63. Delotte J, Barjoan EM, Berrebi A, et al. Obstetric management does not influence vertical transmission of HCV infection: results of the ALHICE group study. J Matern Fetal Neonatal Med 2014;27(7):664–70.
64. Panel on Treatment of Pregnant Women with HIV Infection and Prevention of Perinatal Transmission. Recommendations for Use of Antiretroviral Drugs in Transmission in the United States. Available at: http://aidsinfo.nih.gov/contentfiles/lvguidelines/PerinatalGL.pdf. Accessed May 2, 2020.
65. Department of Health and Human Services. NCCC Launches National Perinatal Hotline. 2004. Available at: https://aidsinfo.nih.gov/news/720/nccc-launches-national-perinatal-hotline. Accessed May 2, 2020.
66. Henrard DR, Phillips JF, Muenz LR, et al. Natural history of HIV-1 cell-free viremia. JAMA 1995;274(7):554–8.
67. Alger LS, Farley JJ, Robinson BA. Interactions of human immunodeficiency virus infection and pregnancy. Obstet Gynecol 1993;82(5):787–96.
68. Joint statement of the American Academy of Pediatrics and the American College of Obstetricians and Gynecologists. Human immunodeficiency virus screening. Pediatrics 1999;104(1 Pt 1):128.
69. Center for Disease Control. Rapid HIV antibody testing during labor and delivery for women of unknown HIV status; a practical guide and model protocol. 2004. Available at: https://stacks.cdc.gov/view/cdc/13256. Accessed May 1, 2020.
70. ACOG Commtitee Opinion No 752. Prenatal and Perinatal Human Immunodeficiency Virus Testing. Obstet Gynecol 2018;132(3):e138–42.
71. Connor EM, Sperling RS, Gelber R, et al. Reduction of maternal-infant transmission of human immunodeficiency virus type 1 with zidovudine treatment.

Pediatric AIDS Clinical Trials Group Protocol 076 Study Group. N Engl J Med 1994;331(18):1173–80.

72. Garcia PM, Kalish LA, Pitt J, et al. Maternal levels of plasma human immunodeficiency virus type 1 RNA and the risk of perinatal transmission. Women and Infants Transmission Study Group. N Engl J Med 1999;341(6):394–402.

73. Balasubramanian R, Lagakos SW. Estimation of the timing of perinatal transmission of HIV. Biometrics 2001;57(4):1048–58.

74. Rachas A, Warszawski J, Le Chenadec J, et al. Does pregnancy affect the early response to cART? AIDS 2013;27(3):357–67.

75. Townsend CL, Byrne L, Cortina-Borja M, et al. Earlier initiation of ART and further decline in mother-to-child HIV transmission rates, 2000-2011. AIDS 2014;28(7):1049–57.

76. Mandelbrot L, Tubiana R, Le Chenadec J, et al. No perinatal HIV-1 transmission from women with effective antiretroviral therapy starting before conception. Clin Infect Dis 2015;61(11):1715–25.

77. Mofenson LM, Lambert JS, Stiehm ER, et al. Risk factors for perinatal transmission of human immunodeficiency virus type 1 in women treated with zidovudine. Pediatric AIDS Clinical Trials Group Study 185 Team. N Engl J Med 1999;341(6):385–93.

78. Riley LE, Greene MF. Elective cesarean delivery to reduce the transmission of HIV. N Engl J Med 1999;340(13):1032–3.

79. Delivery After 40 Weeks of Gestation in Pregnant Women With Well-Controlled Human Immunodeficiency Virus. Obstet Gynecol 2017;130(3):502–10.

80. Scott RK, Chakhtoura N, Burke MM, et al, European Mode of Delivery Collaboration. Elective caesarean-section versus vaginal delivery in prevention of vertical HIV-1 transmission: a randomised clinical trial. Lancet 1999;353(9158):1035–9.

81. International Perinatal HIV Group. The mode of delivery and the risk of vertical transmission of human immunodeficiency virus type 1–a meta-analysis of 15 prospective cohort studies. N Engl J Med 1999;340(13):977–87.

82. ACOG Practice Committee No 751. Labor and Delivery Management of Women With Human Immunodeficiency Virus Infection. Obstet Gynecol 2018;132(3):e131–7.

83. Minkoff H, Burns DN, Landesman S, et al. The relationship of the duration of ruptured membranes to vertical transmission of human immunodeficiency virus. Am J Obstet Gynecol 1995;173(2):585–9.

84. Landesman SH, Kalish LA, Burns DN, et al. Obstetrical factors and the transmission of human immunodeficiency virus type 1 from mother to child. The Women and Infants Transmission Study. N Engl J Med 1996;334(25):1617–23.

85. International Perinatal HIV Group. Duration of ruptured membranes and vertical transmission of HIV-1: a meta-analysis from 15 prospective cohort studies. AIDS 2001;15(3):357–68.

86. Mark S, Murphy KE, Reed S, et al. HIV mother-to-child transmission, mode of delivery, and duration of rupture of membranes: experience in the current era. Infect Dis Obstet Gynecol 2012;2012:267969.

87. Peters H, Byrne L, De Ruiter A, et al. Duration of ruptured membranes and mother-to-child HIV transmission: a prospective population-based surveillance study. BJOG 2016;123(6):975–81.

88. Townsend CL, Cortina-Borja M, Peckham CS, et al. Low rates of mother-to-child transmission of HIV following effective pregnancy interventions in the United Kingdom and Ireland, 2000-2006. AIDS 2008;22(8):973–81.

89. McQuilan G, Kruszon-Moran D, Flagg EW, et al. Prevalence of Herpes Simplex Virus Type 1 and Type 2 in Persons Aged 14-49: United States, 2015-2016. NCHS Data Brief 2018;(304):1–8.
90. World Health Organization. Herpes Simplex Virus. 2020. Available at: https://www.who.int/news-room/fact-sheets/detail/herpes-simplex-virus.   Accessed May 4, 2020.
91. Dickson N, Righarts A, van Roode T, et al. HSV-2 incidence by sex over four age periods to age 38 in a birth cohort. Sex Transm Infect 2014;90(3):243–5.
92. Hollier LM, Wendel GD. Third trimester antiviral prophylaxis for preventing maternal genital herpes simplex virus (HSV) recurrences and neonatal infection. Cochrane Database Syst Rev 2008;(1):CD004946.
93. ACOG Practice Bulletin No 82. Management of herpes in pregnancy. Obstet Gynecol 2007;109(6):1489–98.
94. Cone RW, Hobson AC, Palmer J, et al. Extended duration of herpes simplex virus DNA in genital lesions detected by the polymerase chain reaction. J Infect Dis 1991;164(4):757–60.
95. Boggess KA, Watts DH, Hobson AC, et al. Herpes simplex virus type 2 detection by culture and polymerase chain reaction and relationship to genital symptoms and cervical antibody status during the third trimester of pregnancy. Am J Obstet Gynecol 1997;176(2):443–51.
96. Brown ZA, Wald A, Morrow RA, et al. Effect of serologic status and cesarean delivery on transmission rates of herpes simplex virus from mother to infant. JAMA 2003;289(2):203–9.
97. Brown ZA, Selke S, Zeh J, et al. The acquisition of herpes simplex virus during pregnancy. N Engl J Med 1997;337(8):509–15.
98. Johnston C, Magaret A, Selke S, et al. Herpes simplex virus viremia during primary genital infection. J Infect Dis 2008;198(1):31–4.
99. Prober CG, Sullender WM, Yasukawa LL, et al. Low risk of herpes simplex virus infections in neonates exposed to the virus at the time of vaginal delivery to mothers with recurrent genital herpes simplex virus infections. N Engl J Med 1987;316(5):240–4.
100. Brown ZA, Benedetti J, Ashley R, et al. Neonatal herpes simplex virus infection in relation to asymptomatic maternal infection at the time of labor. N Engl J Med 1991;324(18):1247–52.
101. Fa F, Laup L, Mandelbrot L, et al. Fetal and neonatal abnormalities due to congenital herpes simplex virus infection: a literature review. Prenat Diagn 2020;40(4):408–14.
102. Hutto C, Arvin A, Jacobs R, et al. Intrauterine herpes simplex virus infections. J Pediatr 1987;110(1):97–101.
103. Workowski KA, Bolan GA. Sexually transmitted diseases treatment guidelines, 2015. MMWR Recomm Rep 2015;64(RR-03):1–137.
104. ACOG Practice Bulletin No 220: Management of Genital Herpes in Pregnancy. Obstet Gynecol 2020;135(5):1236–8.
105. Nahmias AJ, Josey WE, Naib ZM, et al. Perinatal risk associated with maternal genital herpes simplex virus infection. Am J Obstet Gynecol 1971;110(6):825–37.
106. Major CA, Towers CV, Lewis DF, et al. Expectant management of preterm premature rupture of membranes complicated by active recurrent genital herpes. Am J Obstet Gynecol 2003;188(6):1551–4 [discussion: 1554–5].

Antenatal Monitoring After Preterm Prelabor Rupture of Membranes

Angela K. Shaddeau, MD, MS, Irina Burd, MD, PhD*

KEYWORDS

- Monitoring • Surveillence • Antepartum • Testing

KEY POINTS

- Preterm prelabor rupture of membranes after viability requires inpatient admission for monitoring of both maternal and fetal status.
- Antepartum monitoring includes close monitoring for signs of intra-amniotic infection, placental abruption, and assurance of fetal well-being.
- Future studies are needed regarding utilization of readily available surveillence technologies to assist in determining which patients for delivery at term versus the late preterm period.

INTRODUCTION AND DEFINITIONS

Preterm prelabor rupture of membranes (PPROM) occurs in approximately 2% to 3% of pregnancies. Management of patients in which PPROM occurs requires careful consideration of multiple factors, including gestational age and risks of expectant management compared with risks of delivery for both mother and fetus. Some prenatal complications associated with PPROM include preterm labor, intra-amniotic infection, placental abruption, and umbilical cord accidents. Given the risk of these significant complications, it is important that a full initial evaluation be performed on these patients to determine if initial signs of infection, abruption, or fetal distress exist. If not, then a comprehensive plan for antepartum monitoring should be formulated if expectant management is deemed appropriate and accepted by patients after thorough counseling.

According to the most recent guidelines from the American College of Obstetricians and Gynecologists (ACOG), published in March 2020, gestational age remains the most important consideration with regard to determining timing of delivery in the absence of a clear indication, such as infection, abruption, or concern for fetal well-

Department of Gynecology and Obstetrics, Division of Maternal-Fetal Medicine, Johns Hopkins University School of Medicine, 600 North Wolfe Street, Phipps 228, Baltimore, MD 21287-4922, USA
* Corresponding author.
E-mail address: iburd@jhmi.edu

Obstet Gynecol Clin N Am 47 (2020) 625–632
https://doi.org/10.1016/j.ogc.2020.08.009
0889-8545/20/© 2020 Elsevier Inc. All rights reserved.

being.[1] Traditionally, PPROM occurring after 34 weeks has been considered an indication for delivery because the risks of expectant management with monitoring were considered to outweigh the risks of delivery and prematurity. A recent meta-analysis of 12 randomized controlled trials, however, found higher rates of neonatal respiratory distress, ventilation requirement, mortality, neonatal intensive care admission, and cesarean delivery in patients undergoing immediate delivery compared with expectant management, with no significant difference in neonatal sepsis rates.[2] The neonatal benefits for expectant management must be balanced with the potential maternal risks. A recent trial specifically evaluating women with PPROM between 34 0/7 and 36 6/7 randomized patients to immediate delivery or expectant management found lower rates of neonatal respiratory distress and mechanical ventilation and no increase in neonatal sepsis in the expectant management group. This trial noted a lower cesarean delivery rate, but had a 2-fold higher rate of maternal complications, including hemorrhage and infection in the expectant management group.[3] Given the results of these recent studies showing neonatal benefits to expectant management, current guidelines from ACOG indicate that either expectant management or immediate delivery are reasonable options with rupture of membranes between 34 0/7 and 36 6/7 weeks after thorough counseling and shared decision making.[1] The decision to manage expectantly requires a detailed plan for antepartum monitoring of both mother and fetus and this monitoring should be performed in an inpatient setting. Rupture of membranes occurring at 37 weeks or beyond is a clear indication for delivery.

PPROM occurring before 37 weeks requires prompt evaluation for signs of overt uterine infection or placental abruption and assessment of fetal well-being to determine if expectant management with antenatal monitoring is appropriate. If expectant management is appropriate, a plan of care for the patient should be established with consideration to gestational age and other concurrent pregnancy complications. Development of this plan should include a discussion with the patient regarding the risks associated with expectant management compared with immediate delivery and the plan for antepartum monitoring of both mother and fetus should expectant management be chosen.

In general, antepartum monitoring in PPROM is performed in an inpatient setting. When PPROM occurs prior to neonatal viability, however, outpatient management and surveillance can be considered after patient counseling and the decision has been made for expectant management. Once the pregnancy reaches a gestational age where neonatal viability is possible, they typically are admitted for inpatient management and monitoring.

The goal of fetal surveillance is prevention of fetal death.[4] With PPROM, there are associated maternal risks, including maternal infection and hemorrhage from placental abruption. Given the significant risk for both maternal and fetal morbidity and mortality, antepartum monitoring in PPROM is of significant importance. This article discusses evidence for fetal and maternal antepartum monitoring modalities in the patient with PPROM and indications for maternal and fetal interventions.

There are important definitions to consider with regard to antepartum monitoring in PPROM. *Antepartum fetal surveillance* is defined as a group of tests and techniques utilized to monitor fetal well-being with the purpose of attempting to prevent fetal death.[4] Two of the most common testing techniques utilized include nonstress tests (NSTs) and biophysical profiles (BPPs). An NST uses a continuous fetal heart rate tracing to identify fetal heart rate accelerations with movement as long as the fetus. This test can exclude fetal acidemia in a neurologically intact fetus. In this test, the fetal heart rate is monitored for a period of at least 20 minutes utilizing an electronic fetal monitor and the results are either reactive or nonreactive. An NST is considered reactive if the fetal heart rate accelerates at least twice by 15 beats per minute for a period of 15 seconds during the 20 minutes. If the gestational age of the fetus is less than 32 weeks, the threshold for reactivity often is lowered to heart rate accelerations of 10 beats per minute for a period of 10 seconds to be considered reactive.[4] A BPP is another common technique utilized for assessing fetal well-being and consists of an NST with the addition of 4 ultrasound markers. These sonographic components include an assessment of amniotic fluid, fetal movement, fetal tone, and fetal breathing. The presence of each component scores a value of 2 points, or 0 points if absent. Each component is defined as follows: the presence of a 2-cm × 2-cm pocket of amniotic fluid, the presence of 3 or more discrete limb or body movements, extension and flexion of a fetal limb or opening and closing of fetal hands, and presence of sustained fetal breathing for 30 seconds or more. If the 4 sonographic components of the BPP are present without the NST component, fetal well-being is considered reassuring.[4]

FETAL AND MATERNAL COMPLICATIONS NECESSITATING ANTENATAL MONITORING AND SURVEILLANCE

Regardless of management strategy, at least half of patients presenting with PPROM deliver within 1 week of ruptured membranes, but the timing of latency from rupture to delivery appears to be inversely related to gestational age at the time of rupture.[1,5] There are both maternal and fetal risks associated with PPROM, necessitating inpatient management in order to facilitate rapid intervention. A common maternal complication associated with PPROM is an intra-amniotic infection, often referred to as chorioamnionitis. Clinically apparent intra-amniotic infection occurs in approximately 15% to 35% of patients with PPROM in the antepartum period and in approximately 15% to 25% of patients in the postpartum period.[1] *Ureaplasma urealyticum*, *Escherichia coli*, *Chlamydia trachomatis*, *Mycoplasma hominis*, and *Enterococcus faecalis* are the most common bacteria associated with PPROM. Rarely, infection can progress to maternal sepsis or death related to maternal infection.

Placental and umbilical cord complications can contribute to poor maternal and fetal outcomes. Placental abruption and subsequent maternal hemorrhage occur in approximately 2% to 5% of pregnancies complicated by PPROM. Umbilical cord compression or prolapse is a common complication that can lead to the need for emergency cesarean delivery or fetal death. Spontaneous intrauterine fetal demise occurs in 1% to 2% of patients who are expectantly managed with PPROM.[1]

Neonatal complications often are identified in pregnancies complicated by PPROM include primarily complications associated with prematurity. These complications can be associated with intra-amniotic infection or placental abruption. Neonates are at increased risk for sepsis, necrotizing enterocolitis, intraventricular hemorrhage, periventricular leukomalacia, and pulmonary hypoplasia. Pulmonary hypoplasia is a significant concern when occurring in the periviable or previable period. These potential complications highlight the importance of admission for inpatient management of these patients.

ANTENATAL ASSESSMENT AND FETAL MONITORING
Initial Evaluation

Management and monitoring of patients who present with PPROM begins at the time of initial evaluation, which includes history, physical examination, and tests to confirm ruptured membranes. The physical examination should include a sterile speculum examination but a digital examination should be avoided. An examination may be indicated if there is a concern for labor. At the time of speculum examination, assessment for pooling of amniotic fluid in the vagina is performed, in addition to assessment of pH of the fluid (often referred to as nitrazine test), and collection of a slide of fluid for microscopic assessment for ferning once the fluid has dried. Amniotic fluid is basic (high pH) and turns nitrazine pH paper blue. Ferning is created when amniotic fluid dries creating an arborization pattern due to the electrolytes present within amniotic fluid. A swab for group B streptococcus culture should be collected at the time of evaluation, prior to starting any antibiotics for latency. Additionally, the fluid is assessed for vaginal bleeding, purulent discharge, or other concerning signs of intra-amniotic infection. A visual assessment of dilation is performed looking for fetal parts or prolapsed umbilical cord that may protrude through the cervix.

A maternal physical examination is performed to identify signs of infection. Vital signs are assessed to ensure absence of fever, normal blood pressure, and pulse. An abdominal examination is performed to assess for any signs of fundal tenderness. Assessment for signs of preterm labor, including subjective discussion with the patient regarding symptoms of abdominal pain, contractions, or vaginal bleeding, is performed and fetal heart rate evaluation is performed with close attention to tocometry to assess for contractions and fetal tachycardia. An ultrasound is performed to determine fetal presentation and to assess the volume of amniotic fluid. Other components to assess for fetal well-being on initial monitoring include the presence of moderate variability on the fetal heart rate tracing, accelerations in the heart rate, and presence or absence of decelerations. If the initial steps of the evaluation and management are concerning for intra-amniotic infection, delivery may be warranted. If after initial evaluation the patient does not have findings concerning for infection and fetal well-being is reassuring, then the patient may be a candidate for expectant management with antepartum monitoring depending on gestational age.

The previable patient with PPROM is the only patient who is considered a candidate for outpatient surveillance and management if this is desired. Prior to discharge for outpatient surveillance, it is recommended that a period of monitoring occur and that the patient have counseling to include the options of immediate delivery by induction or dilation and evacuation or expectant management. If possible, a maternal-fetal medicine consultation and a neonatology consultation should occur to ensure the patient has all of her questions answered prior to making her decision. After this period of monitoring and once counseling has occurred, the patient may be discharged for outpatient management with scheduled follow-up and instructions on when to return. At the time she leaves, she should understand she has an increased risk of infection and placental abruption in addition to her increased risk of preterm labor and fetal demise. She should be made aware that she should return at the first sign of infection to include fevers, abdominal pain or contractions, vaginal bleeding, or purulent vaginal discharge. She should have weekly follow-up to assess for signs of infection. Her plan should include growth ultrasounds at regular intervals and admission at viability for inpatient monitoring at that time.

In the patient with a viable fetus with no signs of infection and reassuring fetal status, admission for inpatient management and antepartum monitoring is recommended. Immediately after diagnosis of PPROM, latency antibiotics are started, a course of betamethasone should be given for fetal lung maturity when appropriate, and magnesium can be considered for fetal neuroprotection. These interventions are discussed elsewhere in this series.

Maternal and Fetal Monitoring and Surveillance

Patients with PPROM should continue to be monitored carefully for signs of impending complications. The patient should have daily physical examinations to monitor for fundal tenderness and close monitoring of vital signs. Serial laboratory tests to evaluate for leukocytosis or other inflammatory markers has not been shown to be beneficial but may help when clinical condition changes. Laboratory tests should be performed with significant vaginal bleeding or concern for abruption. Early findings of infection can be subtle, and providers should have a high index of suspicion in order to detect an evolving intrauterine infection in early stages.

Additionally, fetal heart rate monitoring (NSTs) typically are performed at regular intervals. There is no consensus on the specific interval of monitoring, but most centers monitor at least daily. A recent study comparing various regimens, including continuous electronic fetal monitoring with daily BPP to periodic monitoring with NSTs, 3 times daily, found that patients undergoing continuous monitoring were more likely to have an intervention or cesarean delivery. The study did not find a difference, however, in intrauterine or perinatal mortality.[6] Regardless of chosen interval of monitoring, in the event that a patient has a nonreactive NST, a BPP can be performed to assess fetal status. Additionally, fetal growth ultrasounds should be performed every 3 weeks to 4 weeks to monitor for appropriate interval fetal growth.

An area of interest and research in antepartum monitoring for patients with PPROM has been in surveillance with fetal Dopplers. No large studies have been done to demonstrate the utility of fetal Doppler in patients with PPROM, but several smaller studies have been performed looking at Doppler changes and compared various aspects of pregnancy in patients with PPROM. A study by Carroll and colleagues,[7] in 1995, evaluated Doppler changes in the uteroplacental and fetal circulation. They performed amniocentesis and cordocentesis for microbial culture within 1 hour of Doppler evaluation. The study concluded that there were no differences in doppler values between groups with and without evidence of intra-amniotic infection and that they could not conclude that chorioamnionitis was associated with a significant degree of vasoconstriction based on their data.[7] Shortly thereafter, Yücel and colleagues[8] published a small study in which uterine artery (UA) Dopplers and BPPs were performed on patients with PPROM and the placentas were examined for histologic signs of inflammation after delivery. They found that placentas with microscopically confirmed signs of inflammation were more likely to belong to patients who had abnormal BPP scores and increased systolic-to-diastolic (S/D) ratios on UA Doppler measurement. Based on these findings, they concluded that abnormal BPP scores and elevated S/D ratios on UA Dopplers were associated with impending clinical infection.[8] Aviram and colleagues[9] reported on a larger more contemporary cohort, which included 504 patients with PPROM at a tertiary care center in which they assessed the utility of ultrasound markers for surveillance of patients with PPROM. They found that the median pulsatility index (PI) in the UA doppler was slightly higher in the suspected chorioamnionitis group, but there were similar rates of elevated PI values that were greater than 95% for gestational age. No differences between the 2 groups to other sonographic markers, such as mean amniotic fluid volume, overall BPP scores, or BPP scores less than 6 were identified. Additionally, none of the ultrasound markers was predictive of adverse neonatal outcomes, although neonates in the suspected chorioamnionitis group did have increased rates of adverse outcomes overall.[9] A recent study by Kelleher and colleagues[10] utilized ultrasound doppler technology in a nonhuman primate model to monitor fetal hemodynamics after intra-amniotic inoculation with *Ureaplasma* in addition to assessing the impact of maternal treatment with antibiotics. The study design involved 3 arms: a control group, an intra-amniotic infection (IAI) group, and an IAI group that was treated with azithromycin. Dopplers were assessed in the fetuses, and the UA PI was significantly elevated in the IAI group compared with controls. Treatment with azithromycin restored the values to the levels of the controls.[10] Further studies are needed to assess whether fetal Doppler studies as a marker of fetal infection during expectant management. Additionally, based on the primate study by Kelleher and colleagues,[10] further studies may be warranted investigating therapeutic interventions (eg, continued maternal antibiotics) if early signs of fetal hemodynamic changes are noted on ultrasound without any overt signs of intrauterine infection.

Recommendations concerning the amount of daily activity remains controversial. Given that PPROM is a leading cause of maternal and perinatal morbidity, there is an inclination to question whether bed rest is a reasonable recommendation for these patients in order to prevent potential complications. Antenatal bed rest is widely prescribed in patients with PPROM. Bed rest has not been shown to be beneficial in a variety of obstetric complications and has been associated with increased risk of thromboembolic events and physical deconditioning with resulting muscle atrophy. Two small pilot studies have been recently performed to assess whether bed rest has an effect on latency duration. The first study, performed by Bigelow and colleagues,[11] randomized 36 women to either bed rest or activity without limitation and requiring at least 20 minutes of walking 3 times a day. This study found a decrease in latency that was not statistically significant in the activity group and a "possible" increase in infants diagnosed with necrotizing enterocolitis in the activity group. The second study, performed by Martins and colleagues[12] randomized 32 women with PPROM between 24 weeks and 33 weeks 6 days to complete bed rest (defined as confinement to hospital bed including the requirement to use a bedpan) or activity restriction, which allowed walks on the ward with bathroom privileges. This study found that bed rest did not increase latency to delivery and did not improve maternal or neonatal morbidity.[12] Both of these studies were small, randomized controlled trials. The study by Martins and colleagues[12] utilized the data obtained to calculate a sample size for a randomized control trial. Based on current available evidence, bed rest should not be routinely utilized in the antenatal management of patients with PPROM.

Expectant management with inpatient admission and close antenatal monitoring of mother and fetus is continued as long as the maternal and fetal status remains stable. Certain circumstances necessitate termination of expectant management and monitoring. Evidence of overt intra-amniotic infection as evidenced by maternal or fetal tachycardia, fever, fundal tenderness, or purulent vaginal discharge or amniotic fluid is an indication for delivery in addition to rapid initiation of treatment with antibiotics in order to prevent maternal sepsis. Additionally, new-onset, worsening, or bright red vaginal bleeding should heighten concern for placental abruption and prompt evaluation of fetal status in addition to maternal evaluation. Vaginal bleeding is concerning especially for placental abruption if associated with abdominal pain, contractions, and nonreassuring fetal heart rate pattern. Abnormal coagulation studies with low fibrinogen is strongly suggestive of placental abruption. Antenatal fetal testing showing recurrent fetal heart rate decelerations, persistent fetal tachycardia, or decreased variability may necessitate delivery if unresponsive to intrauterine resuscitative measures. A BPP score of less than 6 of 10 is also suse as an indication to move toward delivery.

SUMMARY

PPROM is a major cause of maternal and perinatal mortality. Given the high risk of morbidity associated with this complication, admission and antepartum monitoring are used to minimize adverse maternal and fetal outcomes. At this time, inpatient antenatal monitoring includes monitoring of maternal vitals and serial examination for signs of infection or placental abruption and daily assessment of fetal status with NSTs. Ultrasound is used to evaluate fetal growth but the utility of Doppler has not been found to be of clear benefit. There is no evidence that bed rest during these admission prolongs latency to delivery or decreases maternal or perinatal morbidity. It is important that providers maintain a high level of suspicion and concern for signs of worsening maternal or fetal status during these admissions that would prompt immediate delivery. Antepartum monitoring of maternal and fetal status is used to determine when delivery should be initiated.

CLINICS CARE POINTS

- PPROM is a complication of pregnancy with a high risk for maternal and fetal morbidity that requires admission and close monitoring after viability.

- Prior to proceeding with expectant management with antepartum surveillance, a thorough evaluation of maternal and fetal status should be performed to rule out infection and ensure fetal well-being.

- Evidence of overt or developing clinical infection, placental abruption, or worsening fetal status should prompt consideration of movement toward delivery.

DISCLOSURE

The authors have nothing to disclose.

REFERENCES

1. Prelabor Rupture of Membranes. ACOG Practice Bulletin No. 217. American College of Obstetricians and Gynecologists. Obstet Gynecol 2020;135:e80–97.
2. Bond DM, Middleton P, Levett KM, et al. Planned early birth versus expectant management for women with preterm prelabour rupture of membranes prior to 37 weeks' gestation for improving pregnancy outcome. Cochrane Database Syst Rev 2017;(3):CD004735.
3. Morris JM, Roberts CL, Bowen JR, et al. Immediate delivery compared with expectant management after preterm prelabour rupture of membranes close to term (PPROMT trial): a randomised controlled trial. PPROMT Collaboration. Lancet 2016;387:444–52.
4. Antepartum Fetal Surveillance. ACOG Practice Bulletin No. 145. American College of Obstetricians and Gynecologists. Obstet Gynecol 2014;124:182–92.
5. Manuck TA, Eller AG, Esplin MS, et al. Outcomes of expectantly managed preterm premature rupture of membranes occurring before 24 weeks of gestation. Obstet Gynecol 2009;114:29–37.
6. Tepper J, Corelli K, Navathe R, et al. A retrospective cohort study of fetal assessment following preterm premature rupture of membranes. Int J Gynecol Obstet 2019;145:83–90.

7. Carroll SG, Papaioannou S, Nicolaides KH. Doppler studies of the placental and fetal circulation in pregnancies with preterm prelabor amniorrhexis. Ultrasound Obstet Gynecol 1995;5:184–8.
8. Yücel N, Yücel O, Yekeler H. The relationship between umbilical artery Doppler findings, fetal biophysical score and placental inflammation in cases of premature rupture of membranes. Acta Obstet Gynecol Scand 1997;76(6):532–5.
9. Aviram A, Quaglietta P, Warshafsky C, et al. Utility of ultrasound assessment in the management of preterm prelabor rupture of the membranes. Ultrasound Obstet Gynecol 2020;55(6):806–18.
10. Kelleher MA, Lee JY, Roberts V, et al. Maternal Azithromycin therapy for Ureaplasma parvum intra-amniotic infection improves fetal hemodynamics in a nonhuman primate model. Am J Obstet Gynecol 2020. S0002-9378(20):30463–4.
11. Bigelow CA, Factor SH, Miller M, et al. Pilot Randomized Controlled Trial to Evaluate the Impact of Bed Rest on Maternal and Fetal Outcomes in Women with Preterm Premature Rupture of the Membranes. Am J Perinatol 2016;33(4):356–63.
12. Martins I, Pereira I, Clode N. A pilot randomized controlled trial of complete bed rest versus activity restriction after preterm premature rupture of the membranes. Eur J Obstet Gynecol Reprod Biol 2019;240:325–9.

SPECIAL TOPICS

Periviable Premature Rupture of Membranes

Kelly S. Gibson, MD*, Kerri Brackney, MD

KEYWORDS

- Periviable birth • Preterm premature rupture of membranes (PPROM) • Latency
- Pulmonary hypoplasia • Antenatal corticosteroids • Amnioinfusion

KEY POINTS

- Periviable deliveries, defined as less than 26 weeks, are a small percentage of deliveries but account for a disproportionately high number of long-term morbidities.
- Premature rupture of membranes in the periviable period occurs during the canicular phase of fetal lung development and may lead to pulmonary hypoplasia.
- Few studies describe outcomes for periviable preterm premature rupture of membranes, and some reports may include only those neonates who received resuscitation.
- Limited data suggest that antibiotics for latency, antenatal corticosteroids for lung maturity, and magnesium sulfate for neuroprotection may be beneficial.
- Amnioinfusion and resealing technologies do not demonstrate clear benefit, but both require further investigation.

INTRODUCTION

Periviable preterm premature rupture of membranes (PPROM), although rare, is associated with potentially devastating maternal, fetal, and neonatal complications. The periviable period, defined as 20 0/7 to 25 6/7 weeks,[1] represents approximately 1 in 200 births, and approximately 80% of those births result from PPROM. Women with periviable PPROM are at risk for chorioamnionitis, hemorrhage, and the psychological and financial consequences of losing a child or raising a child with long-term morbidities. Such morbidities include pulmonary hypoplasia and chronic lung disease, restriction deformities, and other risks of extreme prematurity, such as retinopathy and intraventricular hemorrhage. Because this relatively small percentage of preterm deliveries represents the highest burden on families, it is a logical area of focus because relatively small gains in care can lead to large improvement in outcomes for families.

Few situations in maternal-fetal care are as difficult as counseling near the limits of viability. A majority of providers favor expectant management,[2] but how to safely

Maternal Fetal Medicine, Department of Obstetrics and Gynecology, Case Western Reserve University, The MetroHealth System, Suite G240, 2500 MetroHealth Drive, Cleveland, Ohio 44109, USA
* Corresponding author.
E-mail address: kgibson@metrohealth.org
Twitter: @kellysgibson (K.S.G.)

Obstet Gynecol Clin N Am 47 (2020) 633–651
https://doi.org/10.1016/j.ogc.2020.08.007
0889-8545/20/© 2020 Elsevier Inc. All rights reserved.

achieve the longest latency is unclear. Although the periviable period covers 6 weeks of gestation, the American College of Obstetricians and Gynecologists and the Society for Maternal Fetal Medicine consensus opinion recommend differing interventions based on gestational age throughout the periviable gray zone.[1] Since the original publications on midtrimester premature rupture of membranes (PROM),[3] there have been many advances in obstetrics, including antenatal corticosteroids for fetal lung maturity,[4] the use of magnesium sulfate for neuroprotection[5] and antibiotics for latency,[6] and neonatal interventions.[7] Less established interventions, such as intra-amniotic infusion, resealing agents, and others, are being evaluated for their effects on latency and outcomes (**Box 1**).

This review examines the literature regarding the efficacy of interventions for periviable PPROM. An overview of the diagnosis and initial management of these patients is provided followed by a discussion of the data on traditional and nontraditional treatment options. Given the rarity of this complication, a vast majority of published data are retrospective and included women who were candidates for and opted in for treatment and invention, thus potentially underestimating some morbidities.

BACKGROUND

Extreme preterm birth due to PPROM is associated with high neonatal mortality as well as long-term and short-term severe morbidity.[8] Survival in this periviable period is uncommon and improves week by week. Both survival and intact survival depend on both the age at which membrane rupture occurs and at what gestational age the patient delivers (**Table 1**). Each additional day and week of pregnancy prolongation offers a potential benefit for the fetus.

The etiology for PPROM typically is multifactorial, but all of the factors lead to a weakening of the chorioamniotic membrane. The amnion is composed of 5 layers, including epithelial cells, collagen, a basement membrane, fibroblasts, and an intermediate spongy layer connected to the chorion. The chorion has a matrix of collagen and trophoblastic cells.[9] A weakening of these membranes, either through stretch or collagen degradation, is hypothesized to lead to rupture of membranes.[10]

Many risk factors have been identified for PPROM, although all have a low positive predictive value. These factors include a history of cervical insufficiency or cerclage, antepartum bleeding, multiple gestations, prior PPROM or preterm labor, tobacco smoking, and amniocentesis.[11] Although inflammation from bacterial infection can lead to extracellular matrix weakening, in a review by Kilpatrick and colleagues,[12] infection with gonorrhea, chlamydia, or bacterial vaginosis was not associated with PPROM. This suggests that other bacteria play a role in inflammation as evidenced by a higher level of histologic chorioamnionitis[13] and fetal inflammatory response syndrome.[14]

Box 1
Interventions

Standard interventions
  Antibiotics
  Antenatal corticosteroids
  Magnesium sulfate

Debated interventions
  Tocolysis
  Amnioinfusion
  Resealing techniques

Table 1
Survival by week of gestational age at preterm premature rupture of membranes

	Gestational Age at Preterm Premature Rupture of Membranes					
	20 wk	21 wk	22 wk	23 wk	24 wk	25 wk
Kibel et al,[24] 2016						
Survival	1/88 (12.5) (0.0–35.4)	5/19 (6.5–46.1)	15/31 (48.4) (30.8–66.0)	30/46 (65.2) (51.4–79.0)	—	—
Intact survival	0/8 (0.0) (0.0–0.0)	3/19 (15.8) (0.0–32.2)	8/31 (25.8) (10.4–41.2)	16/46 (34.8) (21.0–48.6)	—	—
Lorthe et al,[25] 2018						
Survival	—	—	12/101 (14.1) (8.2–23.3)	30/95 (39.5) (26.8–53.7)	60/99 (66.8) (56.1–76.1)	99/132 (75.8) (67.7–82.3)
Intact Survival	—	—	9/101 (10.6) (5.6–19.2)	19/94 (29.5) (17.4–45.4)	36/95 (46.8) (34.5–59.6)	76/128 (60.6) (51.8–68.8)
Sorano et al,[26] 2019						
Survival	1/3 (33.3)	7/9 (77.8)	19/23 (82.6)	27/31 (87.1)	—	—
Intact survival	0/3 (0.0)	1/9 (11.1)	3/23 (13.0)	8/31 (25.8)	—	—

Data presented as n/N (percentage) (95% CI).

Regardless of the cause of PPROM, the resultant oligohydramnios disrupts normal fetal development, most significantly in the lungs. Normal lung development encompasses 5 stages: embryonic, pseudoglandular, canalicular, saccular, and alveolar. Periviable PPROM occurs during the late pseudoglandular phase in weeks 8 to 16 or, most often, the canalicular phase in weeks 17 to 28. During the pseudoglandular phase, the segmental bronchi divide into the smaller intrasegmental bronchial tree. The bronchial tree then divides further and develops terminal bronchioles, where the epithelium flattens and type II pneumocytes develop during the canalicular phase. This normal development requires adequate amniotic fluid volume; in the setting of early onset oligohydramnios, the normal development can be disrupted leading to pulmonary hypoplasia.[15,16]

Aside from lung development, periviable PPROM and preterm delivery are associated with multiple other maternal (**Table 2**) and neonatal (**Table 3**) morbidities. Mothers have a higher rate of intra-amniotic infection (9.5%–80.3%), which can progress to endometritis after delivery and potentially sepsis (0%–4.8%). Women are at risk for abruption (4.3%–27.9%) and hemorrhage as well as cesarean delivery (19.3%–68.2%), which often is performed via a classical uterine incision. The rate of neonatal survival varies greatly depending on the gestational age at rupture, the gestational age at delivery, and the institutional practices and parental wishes for resuscitation.[16–26] For example, survival without severe morbidity (including bronchopulmonary dysplasia, severe neurologic injury, or retinopathy of prematurity) in most countries ranges from 20% to 30%; however, in Sorano and colleagues' report from Japan,[26] where neonates are resuscitated at 22 weeks and beyond, the intact survival rate was 63%.

DIAGNOSIS

Rupture of membranes is diagnosed clinically, based on a combination of report of fluid leakage from the vagina and physical examination. The gold standard for

Table 2
Maternal morbidity and mortality after periviable preterm premature rupture of membranes

Study	N	Gestational Age at Preterm Premature Rupture of Membranes (wk)	Intra-amniotic Infection[a]	Abruption[a]	Sepsis[a]	Cesarean Section[a]
Xiao et al,[17] 2000	28	14–28	13 (46.4)	—	—	13 (46.4)
Grisaru-Granovsky et al,[18] 2003	25	16–24	—	—	0 (0.0)	7 (28.0)
Falk et al,[19] 2004	57	14–24	18 (31.6)	—	0 (0.0)	11 (19.3)
Dinsmoor et al,[20] 2004	57	16–24	15 (34.9)	12 (27.9)	—	14 (32.6)
Muris et al,[21] 2007	29	18–24	16 (32.7)	5 (10.2)	1 (2.0)	—
Manuck and Varner,[23] 2014	275	<25	45 (16.4)	29 (10.6)	—	127 (46.2)
Kibel et al,[24] 2016	104	20–24	44 (42.3)	18 (17.3)	5 (4.8)	37 (35.6)
Lorthe et al,[25] 2018	331	23–25	31 (9.5)	14 (4.3)	—	111 (36.6)
Sorano et al,[26] 2019	66	20–24	53 (80.3)	3 (4.5)	1 (1.5)	45 (68.2)

[a] Data presented as number (percentage).

Table 3
Perinatal morbidity and mortality after periviable preterm premature rupture of membranes

Study	N	Gestational Age at Preterm Premature Rupture of Membranes (wk)[a]	Gestational Age at Delivery (wk)[a]	Stillbirth[b]	Neonatal Death[b]	Respiratory Distress Syndrome[b]	Bronchopulmonary Dysplasia[b]	Sepsis[b]	Contractures[b]	Survival (Intact)[b]
Xiao et al,[17] 2000	28	21.6 (2.5)	27.1 (2.1)	—	12 (42.9)	12 (42.9)	8 (17.9)	5 (17.9)	—	16 (57.1) (10 [35.7])
Grisaru-Granovsky et al,[18] 2003	25	22.7 (1.0)	—	—	17 (68.0)	5 (20.0)	—	5 (20.0)	0 (0.0)	8 (32.0) —
Falk et al,[19] 2004	57	20.3 (N/A)	—	30 (52.6)	12 (21.1)	—	—	3 (5.2)	2 (7.4)	15 (26.3) —
Dinsmoor et al,[20] 2004	57	22.0 (N/A)	25.8 (3.4)	13 (22.8)	17 (29.8)	29 (50.9)	8 (14.0)	12 (21.1)	—	27 (47.4) (17 [29.8])
Muris et al,[21] 2007	29	21.1 (N/A)	23.2 (N/A)	—	—	10 (34.5)	—	5 (17.2)	0 (0.0)	12 (41.4) —
Everest et al,[22] 2008	77	19.8 (2.5)	28.4 (3.1)	18 (22.8)	15 (19.0)	36 (45.6)	14 (17.8)	1 (1.3)	—	44 (55.7) —
Manuck and Varner,[23] 2014	275	23.8 (1.2)	26.6 (2.5)	—	46 (16.7)	—	136 (49.5)	111 (40.4)	—	229 (83.3) (67 [24.6])
Kibel et al,[24] 2016	104	22.6 (1.0)	24.8 (2.6)	38 (36.5)	15 (14.4)	—	11 (10.6)	7 (6.7)	11 (10.6)	51 (49.0) (27 [26.0])
Lorthe et al,[25] 2018	331	24 (N/A)	25 (24–28)	17 (6.0)	168 (41.9)	—	29			148 (44.7) (112 [33.8])
Sorano et al,[26] 2019	66	22.7 (0.8)	24.6 (2.0)	—	12 (18.1)	—	34 (63.0)	3 5.6)	2 (3.7)	54 (81.8) (42 [63.6])

a Data presented as mean (standard deviation) or median (interquartile range).
b Data presented as number (percentage).

diagnosis is visualization of pooled amniotic fluid in the vagina. If pooling is not seen on examination, a Valsalva maneuver from the patient may elucidate transcervical leakage. If the diagnosis still is uncertain, vaginal fluid from the posterior fornix may be evaluated under the microscope for arborization (ferning). Arborization, however, is only 69.5% sensitive for detecting amniotic fluid in the vagina between 14 weeks' and 22 weeks' gestation, so PPROM in the second trimester should not be ruled out in the absence of arborization.[27] Likewise, pH in the vagina can be utilized to evaluate vaginal fluid utilizing nitrazine paper but may provide false-negative results in the setting of larger volumes of vaginal discharge, and false-positive results in the presence of alkaline fluids (blood and semen).

Although various commercial kits are available for evaluation of membrane rupture, the risk of inaccurate diagnosis may outweigh the benefit of use in the periviable timeframe. Placental alpha macroglobulin-1 testing (AmniSure [QUIAGEN, Hilden, Germany]) is 94.4 to 98.9% sensitive and 87.5% to 100% specific. Insulin-like growth factors type 1 protein (Actim PROM [Medix Biochemica, Kauniainen, Finland]) is slightly less reliable and is most accurate when performed a short time after membrane rupture occurs, with a sensitivity of 95% to 100% and specificity of 93% to 98%.[28]

Oligohydramnios on ultrasound also may be used to support the diagnosis of PPROM. Caution should be used in utilizing amniotic fluid volume alone for diagnosis of PPROM, however, because no significant difference was found in the mean vertical pocket depth between patients with confirmed term PROM and those with intact membranes.[29]

Intra-amniotic dye installation may be utilized to evaluate equivocal cases of PPROM, although, like amniocentesis, it carries risks of trauma, bleeding, infection, and preterm labor[30] and is limited to cases of a large enough amniotic fluid pocket for instillation. The most well-studied dye agent is indigo carmine, but it is no longer commercially available. Of the alternative dye options available on the market at present, sodium fluorescein may be the safest. The most appropriate dose of sodium fluorescein is not yet established and ranges from 1 mL to 10 mL. Potential maternal side effects include nausea, emesis, anaphylaxis, and transient yellowing of the sclera and palms. No staining of neonatal skin or umbilical cord, placenta, or fetal membranes has been demonstrated.[31] Injection is followed by a speculum examination of the cervix at 15 minutes and 45 minutes postinjection using long-wave UV light to look for yellow-green fluorescent fluid leaking from the cervix.

EVALUATION AND CLINICAL COURSE

Once a diagnosis of PPROM has been established, further evaluation of the patient is warranted (**Fig. 1**). Risk factors for PPROM should be investigated, such as history of cervical insufficiency, vaginal bleeding during pregnancy, multiple gestations, history of spontaneous preterm birth, tobacco use, or cerclage. Chorioamnionitis complicates approximately 35% of patients with spontaneous rupture of membranes at the limit of viability who are managed expectantly,[11] and it may occur before or after the membranes rupture. The highest risk for clinical chorioamnionitis is within the first week of membrane rupture; it drops dramatically thereafter.[32] Close monitoring for chorioamnionitis should continue by monitoring temperature, fetal heart rate, maternal heart rate, fundal tenderness and the development of flulike symptoms. Chorioamnionitis often is associated with preterm labor and delivery and is an indication for delivery, regardless of gestational age. If there is any uncertainty about the presence of chorioamnionitis, an amniocentesis can be considered.

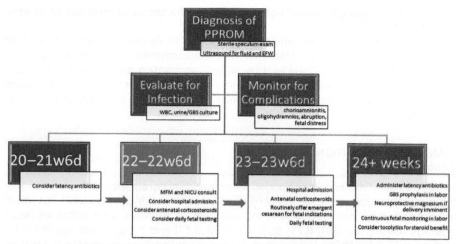

Fig. 1. Decision flowsheet for periviable PPROM. GBS, group B streptococcus; MFM, maternal fetal medicine; NICU, neonatal intensive care unit; WBC, white blood cell count. (*Data from* Raju TN, Mercer BM, Burchfield DJ, Joseph GF Jr. Periviable birth: executive summary of a joint workshop by the Eunice Kennedy Shriver National Institute of Child Health and Human Development, Society for Maternal-Fetal Medicine, American Academy of Pediatrics, and American College of Obstetricians and Gynecologists. J Perinatol. 2014;34(5):333–42.)

Clinical chorioamnionitis has a small but significant risk of progression to maternal sepsis. If chorioamnionitis is identified and managed appropriately with antibiotics and delivery, the risk of sepsis is approximately 5% for pregnancies with rupture of membranes between 10 weeks and 14 weeks,[24] and 1.2% for pregnancies with rupture of membranes between 14 weeks and 23 weeks.[33] Of women with chorioamnionitis, 11% also develop postpartum endometritis. Of all women who experience periviable PROM, up to 40% develop endometritis.[34]

Placental abruption complicates a significant proportion of pregnancies with periviable PPROM and is correlated inversely with gestational age at the time of membrane rupture.[35] Specifically, a study of PROM between 20 weeks and 24 weeks showed a 17% incidence of placental abruption,[24] whereas studies of PROM prior to 20 weeks show a placental abruption rate as high as 50%. In addition to abruption, cord prolapse complicates 1.9% of pregnancies with PROM before or at the limit of viability.[36] Because of the risks of chorioamnionitis, placental abruption, and cord prolapse, most clinicians recommend hospitalization to patients with PROM after the threshold of viability.

Although shorter durations of oligohydramnios may not have a negative impact on neonatal outcome,[37] prolonged oligohydramnios is associated with lower rates of fetal survival and latency as well as higher rates of clinical chorioamnionitis, pulmonary hypoplasia, and emergency cesarean.[38,39]

There has been significant interest in attempting to predict the risk of pulmonary hypoplasia in fetuses affected by midtrimester rupture of membranes. Assessment of the probability of pulmonary hypoplasia could be helpful for both clinical decision making and for counseling of parents. A systematic review and meta-analysis by Van Teeffelen and colleagues[40] evaluated 13 studies and was unable to identify any biometric parameters on ultrasound that reliably predicted pulmonary hypoplasia in these fetuses. Clinically, earlier gestational age at PPROM, latency time between PPROM and delivery, and the amount of amniotic fluid impart higher risks for pulmonary hypoplasia, whereas gestational age at PPROM is the strongest predictor for pulmonary hypoplasia.[41]

Up to 14% of women with periviable PROM eventually stop leaking amniotic fluid from the vagina, and ultrasound demonstrates reaccumulation of intrauterine amniotic fluid.[42] This may be caused by retraction, sliding, contraction, and scarring in the myometrial and decidual layers of the uterus rather than resealing of the membranes themselves.[43] These pregnancies have outcomes similar to those in which PROM never occurred.[42]

STANDARD INTERVENTIONS
Antibiotics

Multiple studies have shown prolonged latency and improved neonatal outcomes with the use of antibiotics in the setting of PPROM after 24 weeks' gestation.[6,44] The use of antibiotics results in a reduction in the numbers of neonates born within 48 hours (average relative risk [RR] 0.71; 95% CI, 0.58–0.87) and 7 days (average RR 0.79; 95% CI, 0.71–0.89).[44] This latency likely is from the antibiotics suppressing or preventing clinically significant intrauterine infections that would lead to delivery. This latency is beneficial at later gestational age; however, its utility in cases of midtrimester PPROM is less clear. To date, no randomized trial has examined antibiotic therapy for PPROM prior to 24 weeks of gestation.

In the absences of a definitive clinical trial, most centers have extrapolated the data from later in pregnancy and treat patients with periviable PPROM with the same antibiotic protocol. As seen in **Table 4**, a majority of studies administered antibiotics, although the regimens varied. In the report by Kibel and colleagues,[24] patients received oral erythromycin, 250 mg, every 6 hours for 10 days. Others used ampicillin and azithromycin[26] or ampicillin and erythromycin,[18] whereas some studies did not report the exact regimen. The use of antibiotics may vary based on gestational age. In the EPIPAGE-2 study, only 81.3% of 22 week neonates had received antibiotics whereas 98% to 100% of 24-week to 25-week neonates had received this treatment.[25]

Although these results are encouraging, they are not enough to definitively guide exact timing, duration, or components of antibiotic therapy. A week of increased latency may allow a fetus on the cusp of viability (22–23 weeks) to reach the threshold set by the local institution; thus, it may be reasonable to treat these patients. For women at earlier gestations, the benefit is far less clear. Furthermore, it is unlikely that the administration of antibiotics weeks after membrane rupture have any additional benefit.

Antenatal Corticosteroids

Approximately 5 decades ago, Liggins and Howie[45] published their sentinel work demonstrating a reduction in respiratory distress in neonates after treatment with antenatal corticosteroids. After several further studies, the National Institutes of Health concluded in 1994 that there was strong evidence that glucocorticoids reduce adverse neonatal outcomes, including death, the respiratory distress syndrome, and other complications, when administered for fetuses between 24 weeks and 34 weeks of gestation.[4] Steroids are thought to induce the type II pneumocytes to increase surfactant production,[46] primarily in the saccular phase of lung development.

As the type II pneumocytes are just beginning to flatten and line the alveoli during the canalicular phase of development in the periviable period, the original studies on steroids excluded patients less than 24 weeks' gestation. As with antibiotics for latency,

Table 4
Standard interventions used for fetal benefit in periviable preterm premature rupture of membranes

Study	N	Gestational Age at Preterm Premature Rupture of Membranes (wk)[a]	Mean Latency (d)[a]	Antibiotics[b]	Antenatal Corticosteroids[b]	Tocolysis[b]	Magnesium Sulfate[b]
Xiao et al,[17] 2000	28	21.6 (2.5)	39.4 (23.9)	25 (89.3)	21 (75.0)	—	N/A
Grisaru-Granovsky et al,[18] 2003	25	22.7 (1.0)	15.6 (N/A)	22 (88.0)	15 (60.0)	3 (12.0)	N/A
Falk et al,[19] 2004	57	20.3 (N/A)	6.0 (N/A)	7 (12.3)	19 (33.3)	4 (7.0)	N/A
Dinsmoor et al,[20] 2004	57	22.0 (N/A)	13.0 (N/A)	37 (64.9)	Yes (N/A)	No	N/A
Muris et al,[21] 2007	29	21.1 (N/A)	14.1 (N/A)	20 (69.4)	8 (28.6)	4 (14.3)	N/A
Everest et al,[22] 2008	77	19.8 (2.5)	55 (33–77)	Yes (N/A)	39 (98)	—	N/A
Manuck and Varner,[23] 2014	275	23.8 (1.2)	20.0 (20.2)	265 (96.5)	272 (98.9)	6 (2.2)	133 (48.4)
Kibel et al,[24] 2016	104	22.6 (1.0)	15.3 (18.3)	Yes (N/A)	Yes (N/A)	—	—
Lorthe et al,[25] 2018	331	24 (N/A)	8.0 (2.8–23.0)	302 (92.8)	210 (68.6)	174 (52.6)	13 (3.9)
Sorano et al,[26] 2019	66	22.7 (0.8)	13.5 (13.0)	Yes (N/A)	Yes (N/A)	Yes (N/A)	—

[a] Data presented as mean (SD) or median (interquartile range).
[b] Data presented as number (percentage); where number was not available, "Yes" was marked if this therapy was in the standard management for patients.

however, a similar trend is observed for antenatal steroid use in the periviable period. As seen in **Table 4**, most institutions did administer steroids. The benefit on survival of these steroids, which are administered only after the fetus reaches the local definition of viability, is not always clear because reaching a viable gestational age also is associated with improved survival.

Few studies have reported on the use of corticosteroids for any periviable deliveries, and those that do report do not specifically separate out the deliveries due to PPROM. A review of neonates born at hospitals in the Eunice Kennedy Shriver National Institute of Child Health and Human Development (NICHD) Neonatal Research Network from 1993 to 2009 reported a significantly low risk of death and neurodevelopmental impairment after 18 months with antenatal corticosteroids at 23 weeks and above.[47] Travers and colleagues[48] performed a follow-up study of the same centers from 2006 to 2014 and similarly found that antenatal exposure to steroids between 22 0/7 and 28 6/7 weeks' gestation was associated with a significantly lower rate of death before discharge and without a higher rate of bronchopulmonary dysplasia or other major adverse pulmonary problems (adjusted RR 0.79 [0.70–0.90] at 22 weeks; 0.68 [0.63–0.74] at 23 weeks; and 0.58 [0.50–0.66] at 24 weeks). Similarly, Mori and colleagues[49] found a significant survival benefit even at 22 weeks to 23 weeks in neonates at 87 tertiary centers in Japan.

Other studies reporting on outcomes of periviable neonates have consistently shown antenatal corticosteroid administration to be of benefit.[50–52] Wapner[53] estimated that 7 to 9 infants needed to be treated to prevent 1 death. Although a specific study on the outcomes for periviable PPROM patients has not yet been completed, these nonrandomized cohorts do suggest a benefit for antenatal corticosteroids as early as 22 weeks' gestation.

Magnesium Sulfate

Of the periviable infants who survive, one of the greatest long-term morbidities is the 8% to 12% risk of cerebral palsy,[54] a group of disorders of development involving movement and posture. Approximately half of cerebral palsy cases are attributed to nonprogressive disturbances that occurred in the developing fetal or infant brain.[55,56] Following observational reports,[57] several large studies evaluated the relationship between cerebral palsy and magnesium administration.[5,58–61] The biologic basis of this effect is thought to be from a reduction in reperfusion injury and free radical damage in neonatal brains after intraventricular hemorrhage.

The clinical trials evaluating the impact of magnesium sulfate on neurodevelopment outcome included women with PPROM but did not evaluate them specifically in regards to their primary outcome. The 3 largest studies to date have suggested a benefit to magnesium sulfate therapy.[62] In 2003, the ActoMgSO4 trial studied 1062 Australian women at risk of delivery prior to 30 weeks. Substantial gross motor dysfunction was significantly less common among children treated with magnesium sulfate (3.4% vs 6.6% [RR 0.51 (0.29–0.91)]).[60] The PREMAG trial, conducted in France and including a 2 year follow-up, found no benefit for cerebral palsy (16.1% vs 20.2%; adjusted odds ratio 0.65 [0.42–1.03]) but did find an improvement in gross motor dysfunction (25.6% vs 30.8%; 0.62 [0.41–0.93]).[61] Finally, the NICHD Maternal-Fetal Medicine Units network conducted the BEAM trial in the United States and found no difference in the primary outcome of cerebral palsy or death (11.3% vs 11.7%; RR 0.97 [0.77–1.23]) but did find a significant reduction in cerebral palsy alone (1.9% vs 3.5%; 0.55 [0.32–0.95]).[5] The primary benefit was in infants born prior to 28 weeks but did not specifically examine those in the periviable period.

In a secondary analysis of the BEAM trial, Manuck and Varner[23] reviewed patients enrolled with periviable PPROM. They found that earlier PPROM was associated with earlier delivery and worse survival. In their regression analysis, treatment with magnesium sulfate was not associated with their composite outcome. Although these limited data do not show a clear benefit for the periviable PPROM patient, a majority of data from infants at 24 weeks and beyond do suggest a reduced risk of death or cerebral palsy with magnesium sulfate (RR 0.85 [0.74–0.98]).[63] Similar to the other established therapies, for periviable deliveries at high risk for adverse neurologic outcomes, magnesium therapy may provide benefit in the periviable period when delivery is imminent.

DEBATED INTERVENTIONS
Tocolysis

Effective tocolysis is an elusive goal in pregnancies with intact membranes. Its role in patients with PPROM is not known. Although tocolysis may offer a few days of pregnancy prolongation, typically for antenatal corticosteroid administration, no treatment has been shown to reduce neonatal morbidity.[64–68] In the periviable period, where each additional day may improve survival, a latency of 48 hours may be clinically relevant. Most studies have a mean gestational age of 28 weeks to 32 weeks, and no studies have been done to examine the role of tocolysis in the periviable PPROM population. As seen in **Table 4**, a majority of centers use tocolysis rarely, if at all, for patients with ruptured membranes.

For patients with intact membranes, a variety of agents have been evaluated for tocolysis, including beta-mimetics, magnesium sulfate, oxytocin receptor antagonists, calcium channel blockers, and cyclooxygenase inhibitors.[64–68] In systemic reviews, there is no evidence of pregnancy prolongation for magnesium sulfate or the oxytocin receptor antagonist atosiban.[64,65] Ritodrine, a β-mimetic, is the only medication approved by the Food and Drug Administration for tocolysis but is no longer commercially available. β-Mimetics have been shown to delay delivery up to 48 hours.[66] Lastly, calcium channel blockers (nifedipine) and cyclooxygenase inhibitors (indomethacin) have been shown to reduce rates of preterm delivery before 37 weeks and reduce the rate of delivery within 48 hours of initiation.[67,68] Although these data could be extrapolated to the periviable period, caution should be taken to apply their findings in the setting of periviable PPROM.

Mackeen and colleagues[69] reviewed 8 studies on tocolysis in the setting of PPROM. A total of 408 women were included, and 7 of the 8 studies compared tocolysis to no tocolysis. They found that, compared with no tocolysis, tocolysis was not associated with a significant effect on perinatal mortality (RR 1.67; 95% CI, 0.85–3.29). Tocolysis was associated with longer latency (mean difference 73.12 hours; 95% CI, 20.21–126.03), but at the expense of lower 5-minute Apgar scores (RR 6.05; 95% CI, 1.65–22.23) and increased need for ventilation in the neonate (RR 2.46; 95% CI, 1.14–5.34). For women with PPROM before 34 weeks, there was a significantly increased risk of chorioamnionitis (RR 1.79; 95% CI, 1.02–3.14) in women who received tocolysis. The numbers were small, but there was no difference in subgroup analysis of different tocolytic therapies.[69]

Thus, although some tocolytics have been associated with increased latency in patients with intact membranes at greater than 24 weeks' gestation, their use in the periviable population is far less studied. Furthermore, there is evidence of potential harm in the form of chorioamnionitis for patients with PPROM. Given the current data, tocolysis for patients with periviable PPROM should be avoided.

Amnioinfusion

Because of the increased risks associated with oligohydramnios in the setting of peri-viable PPROM, amnioinfusion has been proposed as an intervention. It is thought to decrease the risk of pulmonary hypoplasia, limb deformities, chorioamnionitis, placental abruption and fetal death. A 2014 Cochrane review examined 5 randomized controlled trials and found some evidence of benefit to both babies and mothers after PPROM.[70]

Transcervical amnioinfusion improved fetal umbilical artery pH (mean difference 0.11) at delivery and reduced persistent variable decelerations (RR 0.52), but trials were small in size. Transabdominal amnioinfusion showed a reduction in neonatal death (RR 0.30), neonatal sepsis (RR 0.26), pulmonary hypoplasia (RR 0.22), and puerperal sepsis (RR 0.20). One small trial showed a higher likelihood of delivering after 7 days from membrane rupture. Most of these promising findings, however, came from 1 trial with unclear allocation concealment. A Cochrane review concluded that the results are encouraging, but further evidence is required before amnioinfusion for PPROM can be recommended routinely.[70]

Resealing Techniques

Because pregnancies after spontaneous resealing of the membranes have shown normal outcomes, sealing techniques have been proposed to treat PPROM. In addition to allowing the reaccumulation of amniotic fluid, sealing would have the added benefit of a physical barrier against ascending infection.

A 2016 Cochrane review[71] examined 2 studies, which used different techniques. One study compared a cervical adapter (mechanical sealing) to standard care. Although there was no difference between groups for the incidence of neonatal sepsis or chorioamnionitis, the evidence was rated very low quality. Another study compared an oral immunologic membrane sealant to standard care. The immunologic membrane sealant was associated with a reduction in preterm birth (RR 0.48) and a reduction in neonatal death (RR 0.38) but no difference in neonatal sepsis or respiratory distress syndrome. Neither study reported data on overall perinatal mortality.[71]

From these 2 studies, there is insufficient evidence to evaluate sealing techniques for PPROM. Although the immunologic agent has promise, further study is needed with randomized prospective trials. The risks of these techniques still are unclear. Additionally, several cohort studies have been done utilizing other sealing methods, such as intra-amniotic injection of platelets and cryoprecipitate (amniopatch).[72] These techniques also are promising but have not been studied in a randomized prospective manner. At present, none of the sealing methods currently is recommended for routine clinical practice in the setting of PPROM.

SPECIAL CIRCUMSTANCES
Coexistent Cerclage

There is controversy on the management of a cerclage stitch that was placed before the rupture of membranes, which can occur in up to 65% of pregnancies with a cerclage.[73] Although some experts believe that removal of the stitch increases the risk of preterm labor and delivery, others believe that the foreign body may increase maternal and fetal infectious morbidity. Only 1 randomized trial has been performed that examined removal versus retention of the cervical stitch. There was no significant difference between groups in any pregnancy outcome (latency was 56.3% vs 45.8% delivered within 1 week; $P = .59$), but the study was underpowered for analysis.[74]

Several retrospectives studies of PPROM with a cerclage in place have been published.[75–77] No reports found that cerclage retention led to improved fetal outcomes. Ludmir and colleagues[75] reported an increase in neonatal morbidity and sepsis with a retained cerclage. The other studies also demonstrate a trend toward increased pregnancy prolongation but also increased infectious complications with cerclage retention.[76,77]

Because there are no data associating cerclage retention with an improvement in outcomes and there are reported infectious risks with this practice, removal of the cerclage after PPROM is recommended. The best timing of removal has not been determined. Because retention of the cerclage has been associated with latency, leaving the cerclage in place to gain latency for antenatal steroid administration has been proposed. This practice has not been studied, however, especially in the periviable population, so the decision of when to removal a cerclage must weigh the risks and benefits of short-term retention.

Delayed Interval Delivery in Multiples

When a pregnancy with a multiple gestation presents with periviable PPROM of 1 fetus, there is an option to consider delayed-interval delivery of the other fetus(es). Although there is no consensus for an optimal strategy, or a consensus on the best candidates for asynchronous delivery, it seems that periviable pregnancies may be the best candidates, with the most to gain.[78] That said, survival rates are low after delayed-interval delivery after an initial delivery less than 24 weeks.

Delayed-interval delivery is contraindicated in settings with high risk of serious morbidity, such as preeclampsia with severe features, placental abruption, and chorioamnionitis. Amniocentesis to rule out subclinical infection should be considered before offering asynchronous delivery. Maternal morbidity associated with delayed-interval delivery has been reported in up to one-third of women, including endometritis, septic pelvic thrombophlebitis,[79] and severe uterine atony resulting in hysterectomy. One reported noted myometrial microabscesses on pathology after hysterectomy.[80]

If delayed-interval delivery is elected, high ligation of the umbilical cord can be performed with absorbable suture, and the placenta can be left in situ. Postdelivery tocolysis, antibiotic prophylaxis, and cerclage placement has been described but are not well studied and have not yet shown clear benefit. One study showed that most postdelivery morbidity will present within 7 days, so inpatient monitoring may be most useful during this timeframe.[81] This same study concluded that delaying the delivery of the second twin by 2 or more days increased survival from 24% to 56% in the periviable timeframe. At present, asynchronous delivery may be a reasonable option for periviable multiples, but the patient should be counseled about its significant maternal risks. The optimal management strategy is yet to be elucidated.

Preterm Premature Rupture of Membranes After Procedures

Invasive procedures carry with them a risk of membrane rupture, which varies with the type of procedure. Amniocentesis at the limit of viability is complicated by PROM in approximately 1% of cases. These pregnancies have significantly longer latency periods, high rates of rsealing, and higher perinatal survival rates of 91%, compared with 9% in women with spontaneous rupture of membranes at similar gestational ages.[82] Fetal surgery and fetoscopy have higher associated rates of membrane rupture, which may correlate to the number of ports, diameter of ports, location of ports and duration of manipulation.[83] Secondary analysis of the MOMS trial showed that percutaneous fetoscopic meningomyelocele repair dramatically increased the risk of PPROM compared with open repair via maternal laparotomy (91% vs 35%, respectively).[84] Because these leaks tend to be larger, they are less likely to reseal than amniocentesis breaches of the membranes.

DISCUSSION: FUTURE DIRECTIONS FOR STUDY

Many of the recommendations for fetuses in the 22-week to 23-week gestational age range are extrapolated from studies of 24-week and beyond fetuses. The authors recommend further prospective studies in this gestational age group to better elucidate the risks and benefits of the timing for interventions, such as antibiotics to prolong latency, magnesium for neuroprotection, and antenatal corticosteroids. Additionally, larger randomized controlled trials are needed before recommending amnioinfusion or membrane resealing techniques. Such studies should specifically evaluate the composite perinatal and maternal outcomes. Many aspects of delayed interval delivery of multiples would benefit from further study, including identification of its best candidates, determination of the role, type and timing of antibiotic prophylaxis, the role for antenatal testing after delivery of the first fetus, and the risks and benefit of tocolysis.

SUMMARY

PPROM in the periviable period is a major contributor to perinatal morbidity and mortality. Although these deliveries are associated with high risks of fetal and neonatal morbidity and mortality, their low incidence has made studies in this period difficult to complete. Furthermore, when extrapolating from studies done later in pregnancy that may achieve a short latency, the fetus may transition from the previable to the periviable period where survival is possible but with the risk of serious lifelong comorbidities. Families and caregivers must be carefully counseled during this periviable period on the limited data available for interventions and the risks and benefits of each option at each successful week of gestation.

Most data available for periviable PPROM are based on data from 24 weeks and above. These data suggest a benefit for antibiotics for latency, especially when close to viability. Cohort and retrospective studies suggest a benefit for antenatal corticosteroids at 22 weeks and above, when the type II pneumocytes likely are present in fetal lung tissue. Studies for magnesium sulfate to reduce the risk of cerebral palsy and other neurologic morbidities have included pregnancies only at 24 weeks and above. Because periviable neonates are at high risk of morbidity, however, magnesium sulfate's risks likely are outweighed by the potential benefits in the periviable period. Tocolysis and retention of a previously placed cervical cerclage both have been associated with small increased in latency but at the risk of potential increased infectious morbidities. Either should be used with caution in the setting of periviable PPROM. Therapies to increase amniotic fluid or reseal membranes still are considered experimental and should be done only in the setting of research studies.

DISCLOSURE

The authors have nothing to disclose.

REFERENCES

1. American College of Obstetricians and Gynecologists; Society for Maternal-Fetal Medicine. Obstetric Care consensus No. 6: Periviable Birth. Obstet Gynecol 2017;130(4):e187–99.

2. McKenzie F, Tucker Edmonds B. Offering induction of labor for 22-week premature rupture of membranes: a survey of obstetricians. J Perinatol 2015;35(8): 553–7.

3. Taylor J, Garite TJ. Premature rupture of membranes before fetal viability. Obstet Gynecol 1984;64:615–20.

4. NIH Consensus Development Panel on the Effect of Corticosteroids for Fetal Maturation on Perinatal Outcomes. Effect of corticosteroids for fetal maturation on perinatal outcomes. JAMA 1995;273:413–8.

5. Rouse DJ, Hirtz DG, Thom E, et al. A randomized, controlled trial of magnesium sulfate for the prevention of cerebral palsy. N Engl J Med 2008;359(9):895–905.

6. Mercer BM, Miodovnik M, Thurnau GR, et al. Antibiotic therapy for reduction of infant morbidity after preterm premature rupture of the membranes. A randomized controlled trial. National Institute of Child Health and Human Development Maternal-Fetal Medicine Units Network. JAMA 1997;278(12):989–95.

7. Younge N, Goldstein RF, Bann CM, et al. Survival and neurodevelopmental outcomes among periviable infants. Eunice Kennedy Shriver National Institute of Child Health and Human Development Neonatal Research Network. N Engl J Med 2017;376:617–28.

8. World Health Organization. Preterm Birth Facts. Available at: https://www.who.int/news-room/fact-sheets/detail/preterm-birth. Accessed March 8, 2020.

9. Tchirikov M, Schlabritz-Loutsevitch N, Maher J, et al. Mid-trimester preterm premature rupture of membranes (PPROM): etiology, diagnosis, classification, international recommendations of treatment options and outcome. J Perinat Med 2018;46(5):465–88.

10. French JI, McGregor JA. The pathobiology of premature rupture of membranes. Semin Perinatol 1996;20:344–68.

11. Waters TP, Mercer BM. The management of preterm premature rupture of the membranes near the limit of fetal viability. Am J Obstet Gynecol 2009;201(3): 230–40.

12. Kilpatrick SJ, Patil R, Connell J, et al. Risk factors for previable premature rupture of the membranes or advanced cervical dilatation: a case control study. Am J Obstet Gynecol 2006;194:1168–75.

13. Yu H, Wang X, Gao H, et al. Perinatal outcomes of pregnancies complicated by preterm premature rupture of the membranes before 34 weeks of gestation in a tertiary center in China: a retrospective review. Biosci Trends 2015;9:35–41.

14. Romero R, Maymon E, Pacora P, et al. Further observations on the fetal inflammatory response syndrome: a potential homeostatic role for the soluble receptors of tumor necrosis factor alpha. Am J Obstet Gynecol 2000;183:1070–7.

15. Nimrod C, Varela-Gittings F, Machin G, et al. The effect of very prolonged membrane rupture on fetal development. Am J Obstet Gynecol 1984;148:540–3.

16. Winn HN, Chen M, Amon E, et al. Neonatal pulmonary hypoplasia and perinatal mortality in patients with midtrimester rupture of amniotic membranes–a critical analysis. Am J Obstet Gynecol 2000;182:1638–44.

17. Xiao ZH, André P, Lacaze-Masmonteil T, et al. Outcome of premature infants delivered after prolonged premature rupture of membranes before 25 weeks of gestation. Eur J Obstet Gynecol Reprod Biol 2000;90:67–71.

18. Grisaru-Granovsky S, Eitan R, Kaplan M, et al. Expectant management of midtrimester premature rupture of membranes: a plea for limits. J Perinatol 2003; 23:235–9.

19. Falk S, Campbell L, Lee-Parriz A, et al. Expectant management in spontaneous preterm premature rupture of membranes between 14 and 24 weeks' gestation. J Perinatol 2004;24:611–6.
20. Dinsmoor MJ, Bachman R, Haney EI, et al. Outcomes after expectant management of extremely preterm premature rupture of the membranes. Am J Obstet Gynecol 2004;190:183–7.
21. Muris C, Girard B, Creveuil C, et al. Management of premature rupture of membranes before 25 weeks. Eur J Obstet Gynecol Reprod Biol 2007;131:163–8.
22. Everest NJ, Jacobs SE, Davis PG, et al. Outcomes following prolonged preterm premature rupture of the membranes. Arch Dis Child Fetal Neonatal Ed 2008;93: F207–11.
23. Manuck TA, Varner MW. Neonatal and early childhood outcomes following early vs later preterm premature rupture of membranes. Am J Obstet Gynecol 2014; 211(3):308.e1–6.
24. Kibel M, Asztalos E, Barrett J, et al. Outcomes of Pregnancies Complicated by Preterm Premature Rupture of Membranes Between 20 and 24 Weeks of Gestation. Obstet Gynecol 2016;128(2):313–20.
25. Lorthe E, Torchin H, Delorme P, et al. Preterm premature rupture of membranes at 22-25 weeks' gestation: perinatal and 2-year outcomes within a national population-based study (EPIPAGE-2). Am J Obstet Gynecol 2018;219(3): 298.e1-14.
26. Sorano S, Fukuoka M, Kawakami K, et al. Prognosis of preterm premature rupture of membranes between 20 and 24 weeks of gestation: A retrospective cohort study. Eur J Obstet Gynecol Reprod Biol 2019;5:100102.
27. Sugibayashi S, Aeby T, Kim D, et al. Amniotic fluid arborization in the diagnosis of previable preterm rupture of membranes. J Reprod Med 2012;57(3–4):136–40.
28. Marcellin L, Anselem O, Guibourdenche J, et al. Comparison of two bedside tests performed on cervicovaginal fluid to diagnose premature rupture of membranes. J Gynecol Obstet Biol Reprod 2011;40:651.
29. Robson MS, Turner MJ, Stronge JM, et al. Is amniotic fluid quantitation of value in the diagnosis and conservative management of prelabour membrane rupture at term? Br J Obstet Gynaecol 1990;97:324–8.
30. Gibbs RS, Blanco JD. Premature Rupture of the membranes. Obstet Gynecol 1982;60:671–9.
31. Ireland KE, Rodriguez EI, Acosta OM, et al. Intra-amniotic Dye Alternatives for the Diagnosis of Preterm Prelabor Rupture of Membranes. Obstet Gynecol 2017; 129(6):1040–5.
32. Walker MW, Picklesimer AH, Clark RH, et al. Impact of the duration of rupture of membranes on outcomes of premature infants. J Perinatol 2014;34:669–72.
33. Dotters-Katz SK, Panzer A, Grace MR, et al. Maternal Morbidity After Previable Prelabor Rupture of Membranes. Obstet Gynecol 2017;129:101.
34. Moretti M, Sibai BM. Maternal and perinatal outcome of expectant management of premature rupture of membranes in the midtrimester. Am J Obstet Gynecol 1988;159:390–6.
35. Farooqi A, Holmgren PA, Engberg S, et al. Survival and 2-year outcome with expectant management of second-trimester rupture of membranes. Obstet Gynecol 1998;92(6):895.
36. Schucker JL, Mercer BM. Midtrimester premature rupture of the membranes. Semin Perinatol 1996;20(5):389.
37. Kacerovsky M, Vrbacky F, Kutova R, et al. Cervical microbiota in women with preterm prelabor rupture of membranes. PLoS One 2015;10:30126884.

38. Storness-Bliss C, Metcalfe A, Simrose R, et al. Correlation of residual amniotic fluid and perinatal outcomes in periviable preterm premature rupture of membranes. J Obstet Gynaecol Can 2012;34:154–8.

39. Ekin A, Gezer C, Taner CE, et al. Perinatal outcomes in pregnancies with oligohydramnios after preterm premature rupture of membranes. J Matern Fetal Neonatal Med 2015;28:1918–22.

40. Van Teeffelen AS, Van Der Heijden J, Oei SG, et al. Accuracy of imaging parameters in the prediction of lethal pulmonary hypoplasia secondary to mid-trimester prelabor rupture of fetal membranes: a systematic review and meta-analysis. Ultrasound Obstet Gynecol 2012;39(5):495–9.

41. van Teeffelen AS, van der Ham DP, Oei SG, et al. The accuracy of clinical parameters in the prediction of perinatal pulmonary hypoplasia secondary to mid-trimester prelabour rupture of fetal membranes: a meta-analysis. Eur J Obstet Gynecol Reprod Biol 2010;148:3–12.

42. Beydoun SN, Yasin SY. Premature rupture of the membranes before 28 weeks: conservative management. Am J Obstet Gynecol 1986;155(3):471.

43. Behzad F, Dickinson MR, Charlton A, et al. Brief communication: sliding displacement of amnion and chorion following controlled laser wounding suggests a mechanism for short-term sealing of ruptured membranes. Placenta 1994;15: 775–8.

44. Kenyon S, Boulvain M, Neilson JP. Antibiotics for preterm rupture of membranes. Cochrane Database Syst Rev 2013;(12):CD001058.

45. Liggins GC, Howie RN. A controlled trial of antepartum glucocorticoid treatment for prevention of the respiratory distress syndrome in premature infants. Pediatrics 1972;50(4):515–25.

46. Gonzales LW, Ballard PL, Ertsey R, et al. Glucocorticoids and thyroid hormones stimulate biochemical and morphological differentiation of human fetal lung in organ culture. J Clin Endocrinol Metab 1986;62:678–91.

47. Carlo WA, McDonald SA, Fanaroff AA, et al. Association of antenatal corticosteroids with mortality and neurodevelopmental outcomes among infants born at 22 to 25 weeks' gestation. Eunice Kennedy Shriver National Institute of Child Health and Human Development Neonatal Research Network. JAMA 2011;306:2348–58.

48. Travers CP, Carlo WA, McDonald SA, et al. Mortality and pulmonary outcomes of extremely preterm infants exposed to antenatal corticosteroids. Am J Obstet Gynecol 2018;218:130.e1-13.

49. Mori R, Kusuda S, Fujimura M. Antenatal corticosteroids promote survival of extremely preterm infants born at 22 to 23 weeks of gestation. Neonatal Research Network Japan. J Pediatr 2011;159:110–4.e1.

50. Tyson J, Parikh N, Langer J, et al. Intensive care for extreme prematurity—moving beyond gestational age. N Engl J Med 2008;358(16):1672–81.

51. Hayes E, Paul D, Stahl G, et al. Effect of antenatal corticosteroids on survival for neonates born at 23 weeks of gestation. Obstet Gynecol 2008;111(4):921–6.

52. Bader D, Kugelman A, Boyko V, et al. Risk factors and estimation tool for death among extremely premature infants: a national study. Pediatrics 2010;125(4): 696–703.

53. Wapner RJ. Antenatal corticosteroids for periviable birth. Semin Perinatol 2013; 37(6):410–3.

54. Executive Committed for the Definition of Cerebral Palsy. Proposed definition and classification of cerebral palsy, April 2005. Dev Med Child Neurol 2005;47:571–6.

55. Kyser KL, Morriss FH Jr, Bell EF, et al. Improving survival of extremely preterm infants born between 22 and 25 weeks of gestation. Obstet Gynecol 2012;119(4): 795–800.

56. Wood NS, Marlow N, Costeloe K, et al. Neurologic and developmental disability after extremely preterm birth. EPICure Study Group. N Engl J Med 2000;343(6): 378–84.

57. Altman D, Carroli G, Duley L, et al. Magpie Trial Collaboration Group. Do women with pre-eclampsia, and their babies, benefit from magnesium sulphate? The Magpie Trial: a randomized placebo-controlled trial. Lancet 2002;359:1877–90.

58. Mittendorf R, Dambrosia J, Pryde PG, et al. Asssociation between the use of antenatal magnesium sulfate in preterm labor and adverse health outcomes in infants. Am J Obstet Gynecol 2002;186:1111–8.

59. Magpie Trial Follow-up Study Collaborative Group. The Magpie Trial: a randomized trial comparing magnesium sulfate with placebo for pre-eclampsia. Outcome for children at 18 months. BJOG 2007;114:289–99.

60. Crowther CA, Hiller JE, Doyle LW, et al. Australian Collaborative Trial of Magnesium Sulfate (ACTOMgSO4) Collaborative Group. Effect of magnesium sulfate given for neuroprotection before preterm birth: a randomized control trial. JAMA 2003;290:2669–76.

61. Marret S, Marpeau L, Zupan-Simunek V, et al. PREMAG Trial Group. Magnesium sulphate given before very-preterm birth to protect infant brain: the randomized controlled PREMAG trial. BJOG 2007;114:310–8.

62. Chien EK, Gibson KS. Medical and Surgical Interventions Available Before a Periviable Birth. Clin Perinatol 2017;44(2):347–60.

63. Doyle LW, Crowther CA, Middleton P, et al. Magnesium sulphate for women at risk of preterm birth for neuroprotection of the fetus. Cochrane Database Syst Rev 2009;(1):CD004661.

64. Crowther CA, Brown J, McKinlay CJ, et al. Magnesium sulphate for preventing preterm birth in threatened preterm labour. Cochrane Database Syst Rev 2014;(8):CD001060.

65. Flenady V, Reinebrant HE, Liley HG, et al. Oxytocin receptor antagonists for inhibiting preterm labour. Cochrane Database Syst Rev 2014;(6):CD004452.

66. Neilson JP, West HM, Dowswell T. Betamimetics for inhibiting preterm labour. Cochrane Database Syst Rev 2014;(2):CD004352.

67. Flenady V, Wojcieszek AM, Papatsonis DN, et al. Calcium channel blockers for inhibiting preterm labour and birth. Cochrane Database Syst Rev 2014;(6):CD002255.

68. Khanprakob T, Laopaiboon M, Lumbiganon P, et al. Cyclo-oxygenase (COX) inhibitors for preventing preterm labour. Cochrane Database Syst Rev 2012;(10):CD007748.

69. Mackeen AD, Seibel-Seamon J, Muhammad J, et al. Tocolytics for preterm premature rupture of membranes. Cochrane Database Syst Rev 2014;(2):CD007062.

70. Hofmeyr GJ, Eke AC, Lawrie TA. Amnioinfusion for third trimester preterm premature rupture of membranes. Cochrane Database Syst Rev 2014;(3):CD000942.

71. Crowley AE, Grivell RM, Dodd JM. Sealing procedures for preterm prelabour rupture of membranes. Cochrane Database Syst Rev 2016;(7):CD010218.

72. Quintero RA, Morales WJ, Allen M, et al. Treatment of iatrogenic previable premature rupture of membranes with intra-amniotic injection of platelets and cryoprecipitate (amniopatch): preliminary experience. Am J Obstet Gynecol 1999; 181(3):744.

73. Harger JH. Cerclage and cervical insufficiency: an evidence-based analysis. Obstet Gynecol 2002;100(6):1313.

74. Galyean A, Garite TJ, Maurel K, et al. Removal versus retention of cerclage in preterm premature rupture of membranes: a randomized controlled trial. Am J Obstet Gynecol 2014;211:399.e1-7.

75. Ludmir J, Bader T, Chen L, et al. Poor perinatal outcome associated with retained cerclage in patients with premature rupture of membranes. Obstet Gynecol 1994; 84:823–6.

76. Jenkins TM, Berghella V, Shlossman PA, et al. Timing of cerclage removal after preterm premature rupture of membranes: maternal and neonatal outcomes. Am J Obstet Gynecol 2000;183:847–52.

77. McElrath TF, Norwitz ER, Lieberman ES, et al. Perinatal outcome after preterm premature rupture of membranes with in situ cervical cerclage. Am J Obstet Gynecol 2002;187:1147–52.

78. Oyelese Y, Ananth CV, Smulian JC, et al. Delayed interval delivery in twin pregnancies in the United States: Impact on perinatal mortality and morbidity. Am J Obstet Gynecol 2005;192(2):439.

79. Farkouh LJ, Sabin ED, Heyborne KD, et al. Delayed-interval delivery: extended series from a single maternal-fetal medicine practice. Am J Obstet Gynecol 2000;183(6):1499.

80. Roman AS, Fishman S, Fox N, et al. Maternal and neonatal outcomes after delayed-interval delivery of multifetal pregnancies. Am J Perinatol 2011;28(2):91.

81. Zhang J, Hamilton B, Martin J, et al. Delayed interval delivery and infant survival: a population-based study. Am J Obstet Gynecol 2004;191(2):470.

82. Borgida AF, Mills AA, Feldman DM, et al. Outcome of pregnancies complicated by ruptured membranes after genetic amniocentesis. Am J Obstet Gynecol 2000;183(4):937.

83. Gratacos E, Deprest J. Current experience with fetoscopy and the Eurofoetus registry for fetoscopic procedures. Eur J Obstet Gynecol Reprod Biol 2000; 92(1):151.

84. Kabagambe SK, Jensen GW, Chen YJ, et al. Fetal Surgery for Myelomeningocele: A Systematic Review and Meta-Analysis of Outcomes in Fetoscopic versus Open Repair. Fetal Diagn Ther 2018;43(3):161–74.

Unique Considerations

Preterm Prelabor Rupture of Membranes in the Setting of Fetal Surgery and Higher Order Pregnancies

Braxton Forde, MD[a,*], Mounira Habli, MD[b,c]

KEYWORDS

- PPROM • Fetal surgery • Multiple gestation • Fetoscopy • Fetoamniotic shunts
- TTTS

KEY POINTS

- Fetal surgery is a growing field, and one of the primary perioperative complications of fetal surgery is preterm prelabor rupture of membranes (PPROM).
- The PPROM rate in the setting of fetal surgery is related to the surgery performed, the size of the uterine incision/port, the number of uterine ports placed, and the fetal condition being treated.
- Understanding the risks of PPROM in the setting of fetal interventions and the management options will be an increasing important role of the obstetrician.
- Multiple gestations carry an increased risk of PPROM and preterm labor compared with singleton pregnancies.

INTRODUCTION

The 2 most common causes of neonatal death are prematurity and congenital birth defects.[1] Previously, the management of congenital malformations was planned delivery at a tertiary care center with plans for postnatal therapy and intervention. There are now several prenatal interventions ranging from ultrasound-guided procedures to open fetal surgery that have demonstrated improved neonatal outcomes.[2–4] One of the major complications related to fetal interventions is the risk of preterm prelabor rupture of membranes (PPROM) and preterm labor.[5,6] Therefore, balancing the

[a] Division of Maternal-Fetal Medicine, Department of Obstetrics and Gynecology, University of Cincinnati College of Medicine, Medical Sciences Building, Room 4555, 231 Albert Sabin Way, Cincinnati, OH 45267-0526, USA; [b] Division of Maternal-Fetal Medicine, Department of Obstetrics and Gynecology, Good Samaritan Hospital, Cincinnati, OH, USA; [c] Fetal Care Center of Cincinnati, Cincinnati Children's Hospital, Cincinnati, OH, USA
* Corresponding author.
E-mail address: fordebn@ucmail.uc.edu

Obstet Gynecol Clin N Am 47 (2020) 653–669
https://doi.org/10.1016/j.ogc.2020.08.008
0889-8545/20/© 2020 Elsevier Inc. All rights reserved.

maternal risks, neonatal risks, and neonatal benefit is of paramount importance. Even with the noted risks, the benefits for many fetal interventions often outweigh the complications, and offering fetal surgery for a variety of prenatally diagnosed conditions is warranted.[7] Properly identifying and managing the complication of PPROM in the setting of fetal surgery is becoming an increasingly important role of the obstetrician.

UNIQUE CONSIDERATIONS IN THE MECHANISM AND RISK OF PRETERM PRELABOR RUPTURE OF MEMBRANES AFTER FETAL INTERVENTION

Iatrogenic PPROM after fetal surgery typically present as 1 of 2 phenotypes: the "high-leak" PPROM or classic PPROM. Classic PPROM is associated with membrane rupture at the level of the cervix often resulting in labor and an increased risk of chorioamnionitis.[8] High-leak PPROM occurs in the setting of a recent intervention or procedure, where the rupture occurs remote from the cervical os with maintenance of normal amounts of amniotic fluid.[9] Typical tests of PPROM such as ferning, nitrazine test, or pooling may or may not be positive, and the membranes themselves can actually reseal, functionally returning the membranes to a nonruptured state.[10,11] This high-leak PPROM may also transition to a more classic PPROM presentation, with subsequent oligo/anhydramnios, labor, and preterm birth. Interestingly, when the membranes seal off, this does not actually represent the membranes themselves healing, as placental studies have shown persistence of membrane defects in patients who were not even noted to have membrane rupture.[12,13] Furthermore, when histologic evaluation of placentas after fetoscopy is performed, there is minimal proliferation of the chorion and no proliferation of the amnion, but rather proliferation of collagen.[12,13]

The reason for this is likely two-fold. It is important to remember that fetal membranes are both poorly vascularized and not innervated. Therefore, the typical wound healing response, that is, inflammation, fibrosis, and eventually tissue regeneration, does not occur as it normally does in other human tissues.[14] Research on human amniocytes in vitro have noted that the amniocytes may have the ability to repair themselves[15]; however, when fetal membranes have been evaluated in vivo evidence for this has not been present.[16] Likely the most protective mechanism for prevention of PPROM after fetal surgery is not the membranes healing themselves, but rather the strength of the seal between the chorion and amnion.

As mentioned, iatrogenic PPROM after fetal surgery can eventually progress similarly to spontaneous PPROM; however, on the cellular level iatrogenic membrane rupture differs significantly from spontaneous PPROM. Iatrogenic PPROM has been noted to have increased levels of metalloproteinases and decreased levels of lactate dehydrogenase.[17–19] Conversely, interleukin-6 and tumor necrosis factor alpha, known markers of the inflammatory response,[20,21] that have been identified to be associated with classic PPROM have not been identified with iatrogenic membrane rupture.[11] This is consistent with iatrogenic PPROM being due to a mechanical mechanism versus an inflammatory process that precedes rupture.

Even with the knowledge that the defect in the amniotic sac persists after fetal intervention without necessarily causing membrane rupture, there are certain findings that can reflect an increased risk of membrane rupture in the subsequent days. Specifically, chorion-amnion separation,[22,23] an abnormal finding after 16 weeks gestation, can be seen after fetal surgery. Chorion-amnion separation is associated with increased risks of preterm delivery, PPROM, and rarely stillbirth. Thus when a patient is identified to have chorion-amnion separation, closer surveillance is warranted even in the absence of a fetal intervention[24,25] (Fig. 1). There are also procedure-specific membrane rupture risk factors, which will be discussed in detail later.

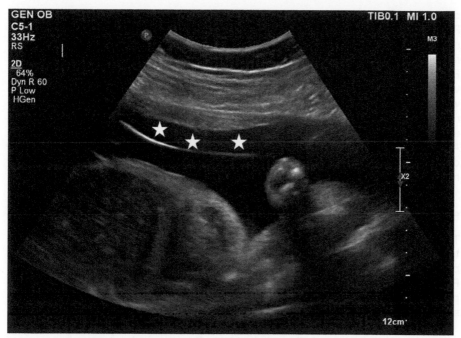

Fig. 1. Chorion-amnion separation. When seen in the setting of fetal intervention, the risk of developing PPROM is high. The chorion-amnion separation is marked with stars.

The greatest risk of iatrogenic PPROM in the setting of fetal intervention is the size of the defect created in the amniotic sac. As expected, defect diameter is correlated with integrity of both the chorion-amnion seal as well as the risk of membrane rupture. It follows that the larger the defect in the amniotic sac, the higher the risk of membrane rupture Significant research in the field of fetoscopy has focused on PPROM. An initial study by Peterson and colleagues found no association when evaluating a cohort of patients undergoing fetoscopy laser and comparing various sheath diameters (2.3, 3.3, 3.5, and 3.8 mm). However, a systematic meta-analysis with data from multiple studies did find a diameter-related risk.[26,27] Beck and colleagues[26] found that the number of ports and more importantly, the maximum diameter of the largest port placed significantly influenced the rate of iatrogenic PPROM and gestational age at delivery. Confirming this, Tchirikov and colleagues[28] noted significantly lower iatrogenic PPROM rates and significantly prolonged pregnancies with the use of 1.2-mm fiberoptic scope through a 2.65-mm sheath versus larger scope and sheath sizes. The specific risks of membrane rupture from fetal surgery are influenced by procedure type as well, which is discussed later.

PRETERM PRELABOR RUPTURE OF MEMBRANES IN THE SETTING OF FETOAMNIOTIC SHUNT PLACEMENT

Fetal interventions for lower urinary tract obstruction (LUTO) or pleural effusions associated with hydrops fetalis is the placement of fetoamniotic shunts.[29,30] The sheath used for fetoamniotic shunts are approximately 13 gauge (1.8 mm) in diameter. In a retrospective cohort of 32 cases of LUTO, the risk of iatrogenic PPROM after shunt placement revealed a PPROM rate of 6% within 28 days of the procedure.[31] In a series of 54 cases of thoracoamniotic shunting for pleural effusions and fetal hydrops the PPROM rate was 15% although the causes for this were believed to be multifactorial.[32] Given the higher rate of polyhydramnios, fetal compromise, and need for more than one shunt insertion in this cohort, these 3 factors could increase the PPROM risk. Other smaller studies have seen similar PPROM rates.[33,34] A recent review of thoracoamniotic shunt placement in 65 fetuses reported a 5% risk of PPROM within 1 week of shunt placement (5%), suggesting the true procedural PPROM-related risk may be lower[31] and more similar to that reported for LUTO. Higher level evidence is needed to truly assess the outcomes associated with amniotic shunting. A randomized controlled trial out of the United Kingdom was attempted but cut short due to difficulty in recruitment.[30,35] Outcomes of PPROM in the setting of shunt placement are shown in **Table 1**.

FETOSCOPIC LASER ABLATION OF PLACENTAL VESSELS

The most common invasive fetal surgery is fetoscopic laser ablation of placental anastomoses for the management of twin-twin transfusion syndrome (TTTS), twin anemia-polycythemia syndrome, and rarely severe selective intrauterine growth restriction. Fetoscopic laser ablation of placental vessels involves the placement of a single percutaneous trocar for uterine access.[37] There does seem to be a significant relationship between trocar size (2.3–4 mm) and risk of membrane rupture.

TTTS itself is associated with an increased risk of membrane rupture associated with polyhydramnios seen in the recipient twin. Snowise and colleagues[6] conducted a prospective cohort study of 154 patients who underwent fetoscopic laser ablation of placental vessels and found an overall PPROM rate of 39% at a mean gestational age of 27 weeks. PPROM occurring after laser therapy significantly decreased the gestational age of delivery, 29 weeks versus 32 weeks, and the average latency from PPROM to delivery by 2 weeks. The time from intervention to PPROM on average was 46 days. Fifty percent of patients who underwent rupture of membranes subsequently delivered within 24 hours. In the analysis Snowise found a significantly increased risk of PPROM with the use of a collagen plug inserted at the end of the

Table 1
Rates of preterm prelabor rupture of membranes in the setting of fetoamniotic shunt placement[30–32,34,36]

Study[a]	Population	N	GA at Surgery (Weeks)	GA at Delivery (Weeks)	Mean Latency to PPROM (Days)	% Cases Complicated by PPROM
Jeong	LUTO	32	17.1	35.5	6	6.3
Picone	Pleural effusions	54	30	36[b]		15
White	Pleural effusions	5	27.4	32.1	5	20
Jeong	Pleural effusions	68	28.3	33.6	<7	4.6
Morris	LUTO	15	20	35.4		20

Abbreviation: GA, gestational age.
 [a] Variable rates of PPROM were reported, as various studies used different parameters for timing of PPROM to be considered perioperative. Jeuong, 28 d; Picone, 7 d; Morris (PPROM <22 wk).
 [b] In surviving fetuses.

procedure. A larger cohort study by Papanna and colleagues[38] found a PPROM rate of 28% postprocedure with a significant risk of delivery before 32 weeks in the setting of PPROM. Others have found an association between preoperative cervical length of less than 25 mm and PPROM with laser therapy.[39,40] Others report an association between the number of placental anastomoses treated and an increased risk of PPROM.[39] The PPROM rate and risk factors for iatrogenic PPROM after fetoscopic laser is an interesting area of future investigation, as a recent study showed that a strong predictor of neonatal survival after surgery was a latency of 28 days or more between surgery and membrane rupture (survival of at least 1 twin in 93% when membrane rupture occurs after 28 days vs 43% before).[40] Further investigation into the natural history of iatrogenic PPROM and prevention strategies to prevent iatrogenic PPROM in the setting of fetoscopic laser ablation of placental vessels is warranted. Outcomes of PPROM in the setting of fetoscopic laser ablation of placental vessels are shown in **Table 2**.

RADIOFREQUENCY ABLATION

Twin reversed arterial perfusion (TRAP) is a rare but potentially lethal disease, affecting roughly 1 in 35,000 pregnancies and 1 in 100 monozygotic twin pregnancies.[43] A full review is beyond the scope of this article, but it is characterized by a normal twin and an acardiac twin (perfused by the cardiac twin) that is sustained through placental anastomoses. The cardiac or "pump" twin is thus at risk for development of hydrops and other complications due to high-output cardiac failure.[44] There are several treatments if intervention is required to protect the pump twin; however, the most common intervention is radiofrequency ablation (RFA). RFA can also be used for selective reduction in the setting of advanced twin-twin transfusion or other abnormalities of higher order pregnancies.[45] RFA involves generating heat by using alternating current at frequencies between 200 and 1200 kHz between the ablation needle and grounding pad. The high temperatures coagulate the target vessels.[46]

There are only a few series reviewing RFA for selective fetal reduction; however, the data that exist are promising. Livingston and colleagues[47] found a PPROM rate of 6% when RFA was used for TRAP at an average gestational age of 21 weeks. Lee and colleagues[48] reported on a larger cohort of TRAP sequence twins (29) finding higher PPROM rates but had similar gestational age at delivery of greater than or equal to

Table 2
Rates of preterm prelabor rupture of membranes in the setting of fetoscopic laser ablation of placental anastomoses[6,38–42]

Study	Population	N	GA at Surgery (Weeks)	GA at Delivery (Weeks)	Median Latency to PPROM (Days)	PPROM <34 wk	Median Latency from PPROM to Delivery (Days)	% Cases Complicated by PPROM
Snowise	TTTS	154	20.7	31.2	46	NS	1	39
Papanna	TTTS	487	20.8	31.2	NS	NS	NS	28
Malshe[a]	TTTS	203	20.6	30.9	NS	80	NS	39
Ruegg	TTTS	39	20.3	31.5	57	NS	3	43
Habli	TTTS	154	21	31	41	NS	NS	27

Abbreviation: GA, gestational age.
[a] Includes the Snowise cohort.

35 weeks. Lee also reviewed the North American Fetal Therapy Network's Registry data and again found high levels of success with a median gestational age at delivery of 37 weeks.[49] Paramasivam and colleagues[45] examined RFA use during selective reduction with TTTS and found similar results. They reported a PPROM rate of 14% and a gestational age at delivery of 36 weeks.[45] RFA, even with the risks of high tissue temperatures, has been shown to be an effective fetal intervention with excellent gestational age outcomes at delivery and PPROM rates. The overall success is thought to be due to the small diameter of the ablation device and single uterine entry. Outcomes regarding PPROM in the setting of RFA are presented in **Table 3**.

FETOSCOPIC MYELOMENINGOCELE REPAIR

Because of the significant obstetric and maternal complications associated with open fetal surgery, an emerging technique for the repair of fetal myelomeningocele (MMC) was developed—fetoscopic MMC repair.[50–53] Initial attempts were associated with significant variations in approach, percutaneous versus laparotomy, and the number of ports for uterine access, 2 versus 3 ports. A recent meta-analysis by Kabagambe and colleagues[54] demonstrated no significant difference in combined fetal and post-natal mortality between fetoscopic and open repair and no significant difference in postnatal ventricular shunt placement. This has resulted in an increase in the feto-scopic repair approach and will likely become more commonplace.

The most significant technique variations affecting PPROM revolve around the absence or presence of maternal laparotomy to access the uterus. Percutaneous MMC repair is associated with almost universal membrane rupture (96%); however, the use of a laparotomy with fetoscopic uterine entry decreased the PPROM rate to that of an open technique, if not less.[55] The true PPROM risk is still uncertain, as the total number of cases of fetoscopic MMC repair cases is still limited. However, Belfort and colleagues[56] reported a PPROM rate of 1/10 patients with fetoscopic repair compared with 4/12 with open repair. The maternal comorbidity was signifi-cantly less with fetoscopic MMC repair, from lower hemorrhage risk related to smaller uterine defect. The smaller uterine defect may have additional significance in future pregnancies. Vaginal delivery is the recommended mode of delivery after fetoscopic procedures unless maternal or neonatal condition necessitates cesarean delivery. Outcomes regarding PPROM in the setting of various studies of fetoscopic MMC repair are presented in **Table 4**.

FETOSCOPIC TRACHEAL BALLOON OCCLUSION FOR CONGENITAL DIAPHRAGMATIC HERNIAS

Interventions are under evaluation for in utero treatment of congenital diaphragmatic hernias. The natural history and postnatal treatment of congenital diaphragmatic her-nia is beyond the scope of this review; however, congenital diaphragmatic hernia is a well-known cause of severe neonatal morbidity or mortality.[61,62] A prenatally measured observed/expected lung/head ratio less than 25% and intrathoracic liver herniation identifies patients considered to have a high perinatal mortality rates.[63] Even with extracorporeal membrane oxygen the mortality rates remain high. An emerging and interesting therapy to reduce the rate of severe congenital pulmonary hypertension is fetoscopic endoluminal tracheal occlusion (FETO).[64,65] This procedure is typically performed in the late second trimester. The size of the sheath for this pro-cedure is 3 mm.

As one would expect, FETO is associated with an increased PPROM risk. The largest study to date was a multicenter trial with a PPROM rate of 47% and a median

Table 3

Rates of preterm prelabor rupture of membranes in the setting of radiofrequency ablation for selective reduction in the setting of twin reversed arterial perfusion or twin-twin transfusion syndrome[45,47,48]

Study	Population	N	GA at Surgery (Weeks)	GA at Delivery (Weeks)	Median Latency to PPROM (Days)	Median Latency from PPROM to Delivery (Days)	% Cases Complicated by PPROM
Livingston	TRAP	17	21	37	35	NS	6
Paramasivam	TTTS	35	17.6	36	56	NS	14
Lee	TRAP	29	18–24	35	NS	NS	17

Abbreviation: GA, gestational age.

Table 4
Rates of preterm prelabor rupture of membranes in the setting of percutaneous or open fetoscopic myelomeningocele repair[53,56–60]

Study	Population	N	GA at Surgery (Weeks)	GA at Delivery (Weeks)	Mean Latency to PPROM (Days)	% Cases Complicated by PPROM
Graf	MMC Percutaneous	71	22.5	32.2	NS	NS
Pedreira	MMC Percutaneous	32	26.7	32.4	29	84
Pedreira	MMC Percutaneous	13	26.9	33.7	25	69
Degenhardt	MMC Percutaneous	51	24	33	40	84
Verbeek	MMC Percutaneous	19	23	32	NS	85
Belfort	MMC Ex-lap	28	25	36	NS	36
Cortes	MMC Ex-lap	32	25	38	NS	NS

Abbreviations: Ex-lap, exploratory laparotomy; GA, gestational age.

time to rupture of 30 days.[66] Subsequent trials have shown similar rates of PPROM.[67] Operative time has been shown to correlate with PPROM risk in the setting of FETO, and longer operative times are associated with shorter interval to PPROM.[66] PPROM in the setting of FETO significantly increases the risk of early preterm birth. Interestingly, however, these neonates delivering before 32 to 34 weeks still had less morbidity than their nonintervention counterparts. Of note, it is important to assess balloon status at the time of PPROM diagnosis. The balloon is typically deflated at 34 weeks. If the balloon is still in place, it must be decompressed before delivery via ultrasound guidance, or if delivery is imminent, an Ex Utero Intrapartum Treatment (EXIT) procedure should be performed for fetal airway management so that the balloon can be removed for neonatal ventilation. If a patient has had the balloon decompressed or removed and subsequently experiences PPROM, vaginal delivery is an option. Outcomes regarding PPROM and FETO are presented in **Table 5**.

PRETERM PRELABOR RUPTURE OF MEMBRANES IN THE SETTING OF OPEN FETAL SURGERY

Open fetal surgery has been used to treat several fetal abnormalities. Because of the high maternal and fetal risks, many of those treatments are no longer performed. One

Table 5
Rates of preterm prelabor rupture of membranes in the setting of fetoscopic tracheal occlusion for severe fetal congenital diaphragmatic hernia[66,67]

Study	Population	N	GA at Surgery (Weeks)	GA at Delivery (Weeks)	Median Latency to PPROM (Days)	% Cases Complicated by PPROM
Jani	FETO	210	27.1	35.3	30	47
Baschat	FETO	21	28.5	36.1	NS	24

Abbreviation: GA, gestational age.

of the primary risks with open fetal surgery is the risk of membrane rupture leading pre-term delivery. The total causes of high rate of membrane rupture is likely multifactorial but the main risks of membrane rupture are likely due to the size of hysterotomy (6–8 cm) as well as the predisposition for contractions postoperatively.[68,69]

Open fetal surgery for MMC repair is the most studied of all of these prenatal inter-ventions. In a multicenter, randomized controlled trial (Management of Myelomeningo-cele Study) comparing prenatal and postnatal MMC repair, 78 fetuses underwent prenatal repair of MMC with a 46% PPROM compared with 8% undergoing postnatal repair.[68] A subsequent large retrospective cohort study from Brazil found lower rates of PPROM (27%). This may have been related to selection bias but may also be related to surgical technique. The Brazilian group was unable to use the uterine stapler and thus used a different technique on the uterus.[70,71] Additionally, their criteria for surgery included later gestations, which may have impacted the PPROM rates. Further inves-tigation into their surgical technique is needed to see if the PPROM rate can be repro-duced. Minimizing iatrogenic PPROM after open fetal surgery may reopen open fetal surgery as a more viable surgical technique for various prenatal interventions.

The management and natural course of iatrogenic PPROM after open fetal surgery has typically followed standard PPROM care. Data regarding the latency from PPROM and subsequent delivery are limited. The management of patients in the setting of open fetal surgery tends to be complicated by the uterine incision, which has a high rate of dehiscence and thus may lead to earlier delivery via cesarean when uterine contractions are identified (as opposed to PPROM in the setting of fetoscopic sur-gery). What is known regarding risks for PPROM after open fetal surgery is that chorion-amnion separation identified postoperatively conveys a high risk of subse-quent PPROM (59% vs only 21% of patients without chorion amnion separation).[23]

INTERVENTIONS TO TREAT OR PREVENT PRETERM PRELABOR RUPTURE OF MEMBRANES IN THE SETTING OF FETAL SURGERY

Multiple techniques have been studied to either induce membrane sealing or prevent membrane rupture in the setting of fetal surgery in animal models; however, one of the only techniques that has been applied clinically is the insertion of a collagen plug. A small uncontrolled study by Chang and colleagues[72] reported on a very meticulous technique for collagen plug and port insertion with very low rates (4.2%) of PPROM in twins undergoing fetoscopic laser for TTTS. However, this has not been replicated. In a larger study by Papanna and colleagues,[41] the investigators found no difference in PPROM rates between TTTS patients who underwent surgical management with or without a collagen plug. As previously mentioned, Snowise found an increased risk of PPROM in the setting of fetoscopic laser when a collagen plug was used.[6] In the largest study of its kind, Engels and colleagues found no statistically significant differ-ence in PPROM rates in patients who underwent FETO for congenital diaphragmatic hernia (CDH) when a collagen plug was or was not used (48 vs 39%, respectively) with a nonsignificant trend toward membrane rupture.[73] Given the results of these studies, collagen plugs have not been recommended for prevention of PPROM in the setting of fetoscopy.

Another technique for membrane repair is the amniopatch first described by Quin-tero and colleagues[74] in 1996. It consists of infusing a platelet concentrate and cryo-precipitate into the amniotic cavity. Platelet activation and fibrin deposition leads to formation of a plug to seal the defect site. The reported success rate of amniopatch varies widely, from 10% to 60%,[75–77] with much higher rates of membrane sealing in the setting of iatrogenic membrane rupture. A randomized controlled trial of 100 patients who had spontaneous membrane rupture randomized the use of amniopatch in patients receiving standard therapy with antibiotics/corticosteroids. This study found that amniopatch was successful in sealing of the membrane defect in 12% of the intervention group, with 0% of patients in the control group. Furthermore, in the amniopatch group, 24% of patients had restoration of normal amniotic fluid index (although half of these patients' normalization was transient, only 12% of total patients had sealing of the membrane defect).[78] Given, however, the low number of resealing, it is unclear if neonatal benefit is conferred. There is limited information related to the use of amniopatch for iatrogenic PPROM. A recent study by Chmait and colleagues looked specifically at patients who underwent PPROM within 15 days of fetoscopic laser for twin-twin transfusion. Amniopatch was successful in 12/19 patients, with improved gestational age at delivery (35 vs 28 weeks) and improved 30-day survival in the recipient twin (100% vs 57%).[79–84]

OTHER UNIQUE CONSIDERATIONS—PRETERM PRELABOR RUPTURE OF MEMBRANES IN THE SETTING OF MULTIPLE GESTATION

It is of particular importance to understand PPROM in the setting of multiple gestation in the absence of interventions to be able to understand procedure-related risk. The frequency of PPROM is higher in multifetal gestations.[85,86] A large population study by Pakrashi and colleagues reported the complication of PPROM occurs in 11% of twins, 19% of triplets, and 20% of quadruplets.[86] Mercer and colleagues[85] found PPROM rates in twins at roughly 7% to 8%, which still would be double the rate of PPROM in singleton pregnancies. These studies also further highlighted the earlier timing of PPROM in the setting of multiple gestation, with 36% of twin PPROM, 28% of triplet PPROM, and 50% of quadruplet PPROM occurring at less than 28 weeks.

The data regarding the natural course and history of PPROM with multiple gestations are limited. However, some retrospective studies have demonstrated trends. A study by Trentacoste and colleagues evaluated membrane rupture in the setting of

Table 6
Rates of preterm prelabor rupture of membranes in the setting of multiple gestation[86–90,100,101]

Study	Population	N	GA at PPROM (Weeks)	Median Latency (Days)	Latency >7 d %	P
Mercer	Twin	99	30.1	3.6	9%	NS
	Control	99	30.6	4.1	10%	
Bianco	Twin	116	32.4	0.1	7%	NS
	Control	116	32.2	0.8	6%	
Myles	Twin	28	29.5	4.3	n/a	
	Control	119	30.0	8.6	n/a	
Hsieh	Twin	48	29.7	3.4	8%	n/a
	Control	131	30.8	4.4	15%	
Jacquemyn	Twin	33		0.8	11%	0.06
	Control	66		2.0	23%	
Trentacoste	Twin	49 n/a	31	0	22%	n/a
	Control					

Abbreviation: GA, gestational age.

dichorionic diamniotic twin gestation before 34 weeks. This study indicated that the median gestational age at the time of membrane rupture was 31 weeks with a median latency of less than 1 day. Only 22.4% of patients had a latency of 7 days or more.[87] Interestingly, PPROM less than 30 weeks was associated with significantly higher rates of latency of 7 or more days (47.1% vs 9.4%) compared with PPROM after 30 weeks gestational age. Earlier studies have found similar findings, with the mean gestational age at the time of delivery being roughly 30 to 32 weeks.[88–99] These earlier studies also noted a shorter latency period, with anywhere from 7% to 22% of twins having a latency of 7 or more days. Outcomes regarding PPROM in the setting of multiple gestation are presented in **Table 6**.

CLINICS CARE POINTS

- The amniotic sac does not heal in the same fashion as normal tissue due to absence of innervation and blood supply.
- Chorion-amnion separation after 16 weeks is an abnormal finding and when seen after fetal intervention, is associated with a high risk of membrane rupture.
- PPROM rates in the setting of fetoamniotic shunt placement are associated with the number of procedures performed and the indication. Thoracoamniotic shunts are associated with higher rates of PPROM.
- Collagen plugs inserted at the end of a fetoscopic laser surgery have been associated with increased PPROM rates.
- RFA is a very well-tolerated surgery for selective reduction and portends a lower PPROM risk than previously performed surgeries such as bipolar coagulation of the cord.
- Fetoscopic MMC repair is an emerging technique that is replacing open fetal MMC repairs due to similar neonatal outcomes but improved maternal outcomes.
- Vaginal delivery is an option in individuals undergoing fetoscopic procedures.
- Fetoscopic tracheal balloon occlusion seems to improve outcomes in severe congenital CDH; however, it carries a high risk of PPROM as well as preterm delivery.
- The balloon used for FETO must be deflated before delivery, either through needle decompression under US guidance, removal via repeat fetoscopy, or via EXIT to secure the airway.
- Open fetal surgery is becoming less common due to improvements in fetoscopic surgery; however, newer techniques may lower the PPROM rate and will continue to make open fetal surgery a relevant operative technique.
- Amniopatch, when successful, can significantly prolong latency after iatrogenic PPROM, but the overall success rate is relatively low.
- Multiple gestations carry at least twice the risk of PPROM compared with singleton pregnancies.

REFERENCES

1. Hoyert DL, Xu J. Deaths: preliminary data for 2011. Natl Vital Stat Rep 2012; 61(6):1–51. Available at: http://www.cdc.gov/nchs/data/nvsr/nvsr61/nvsr61_06. pdf (PDF - 891 KB. Accessed July 23, 2013.

2. Maselli KM, Badillo A. Advances in fetal surgery. Ann Transl Med 2016; 4(20):394.

3. Garabedian C, Jouannic JM, Benachi A, et al. Fetal therapy and fetoscopy: A reality in clinical practice in 2015. J Gynecol Obstet Biol Reprod 2015;44(7): 597–604.

4. Deprest JA, Devlieger R, Srisupundit K, et al. Fetal surgery is a clinical reality. Semin Fetal Neonatal Med 2010;16(1):58–67.

5. Farmer D. Fetal surgery. BMJ 2003;326(7387):461–2.

6. Snowise S, Mann LK, Moise KJ, et al. Preterm prelabor rupture of membranes after fetoscopic laser surgery for twin-twin transfusion syndrome. Ultrasound Obstet Gynecol 2017;49(5):607–11.

7. Committee on Obstetric Practice, Society for Maternal-Fetal Medicine. Committee Opinion No. 720: Maternal-Fetal Surgery for Myelomeningocele. Obstet Gynecol 2017;130(3):164–7.

8. Committee on Practice Bulletins-Obstetrics. ACOG Practice Bulletin No 188. Prelabor Rupture of Membranes. Obstet Gynecol 2018;131(1):1–14.

9. Tchirikov M, Schlabritz-Loutsevitch N, Maher J, et al. Mid-trimester preterm premature rupture of membranes (PPROM): etiology, diagnosis, classification, international recommendations of treatment options and outcome. J Perinatal Med 2017;46(5):465–88.

10. Kishida T, Negishi H, Sagawa T, et al. Spontaneous reseal of the fetal membranes in patients with high-leak PROM, confirmed by intra-amniotic injection of a dye (phenol-sulfonphthalein). Eur J Obstet Gynecol Reprod Biol 1996; 68(1):219–21.

11. Devlieger R, Millar LK, Bryant-Greenwood G, et al. Fetal membrane healing after spontaneous and iatrogenic membrane rupture: a review of current evidence. Am J Obstet Gynecol 2006;195(6):1512–20.

12. Gratacos E, Sanin-Blair J, Lewi L, et al. A histological study of fetoscopic membrane defects to document membrane healing. Placenta 2006;27:452–6.

13. Carvalho NS, Moron AF, Menon R, et al. Histological evidence of reparative activity in chorioamniotic membrane following open fetal surgery for myelomeningocele. Exp Ther Med 2017;14(4):3732–6.

14. Singer AJ, Clark RA. Cutaneous wound healing. N Engl J Med 1999;341(10): 738–46.

15. Quintero RA, Carreno CA, Yelian F, et al. kinetics of amnion cells after microsurgical injury. Fetal Diagn Ther 1996;11:348–56.

16. Devlieger R, Gratacós E, Wu J, et al. J.A. DeprestAn organ-culture for in vitro evaluation of fetal membrane healing capacity. Eur J Obstet Gynecol Reprod Biol 2000;92:145–50.

17. Devlieger R, Riley SC, Verbist L, et al. Matrix metalloproteinases-2 and −9 and their endogenous tissue inhibitors in tissue remodeling after sealing of the fetal membranes in a sheep model of fetoscopic surgery. J Soc Gynecol Investig 2002;9:137–45.

18. Devlieger R, Deprest JA, Gratacós E, et al. Matrix metalloproteinases −2 and −9 and their endogenous tissue inhibitors in fetal membrane repair following fetoscopy in a rabbit model. Mol Hum Reprod 2000;6:479–85.

19. Papanna R, Mann LK, Moise KJ Jr, et al. Histologic changes of the fetal membranes after fetoscopic laser surgery for twin-twin transfusion syndrome. Pediatr Res 2015;78:247–55.

20. Wang XJ, Li L, Cui SH. Role of collagen III, CTGF and TNF-alpha in premature rupture of human fetal membranes (original in Chinese). Sichuan Da Xue Xue Bao Yi Xue Ban 2009;40(4):658–61.

21. Hatzidaki E, Gourguitis D, Manoura A, et al. Interleukin-6 in preterm premature rupture of membranes as an indicator of neonatal outcome. Acta Obstet Gynecol Scand 2005;84(7):632–8.

22. Sydorak R, Hirose S, Sandberg P, et al. Chorioamniotic membrane separation following fetal surgery. J Perinatol 2002;22:407–10.

23. Soni S, Moldenhaur JS, Spinner SS, et al. Chorioamniotic membrane separation and preterm premature rupture of membranes complicating in utero myelomeningocele repair. Am J Obstet Gynecol 2016;214(5):647.e1-7.

24. Bibbo C, Little SE, Bsat J, et al. Chorioamniotic separation found on obstetric ultrasound and perinatal outcome. AJP Rep 2016;6(3):e337–43.

25. Ortiz JU, Eixarch E, Peguero A, et al. Chorioamniotic membrane separation after fetoscopy in monochorionic twin pregnancy: incidence and impact on perinatal outcome. Ultrasound Obstet Gynecol 2016;47(3):345–9.

26. Beck V, Lewi P, Gucciardo L, et al. Preterm prelabor rupture of membranes and fetal survival after minimally invasive fetal surgery: a systematic review of the literature. Fetal Diagn Ther 2012;31:1–9.

27. Petersen S, Doné E, Gardener G, et al: Rate of amniorrhexis is not influenced by fetoscopic cannula diameter: 19th World Congress on Ultrasound in Obstetrics and Gynecology, Hamburg 2009.

28. Tchirikov M, Oshovskyy V, Steetskamp J, et al. Neonatal outcome using ultrathin fetoscope for laser coagulation in twin-to-twin-transfusion syndrome. J Perinat Med 2001;39(6):725–30.

29. Gregory C, Wright J, Schwartz RL. A review of Fetal thoracoamniotic and vesicoamniotic shunt procedures. J Obstet Gynecol Neonatal Nurs 2012;41(3):426–33.

30. Morris RK, Khan KS, Kilby MD. Vesicoamniotic shunting for fetal lower urinary tract obstruction: an overview. Arch Dis Child Fetal Neonatal Ed 2007;92(3):F166–8.

31. Jeong BD, Won HS, Lee MY. Perinatal outcomes of fetal lower urinary tract obstruction after vesicoamniotic shunting using a double-basket catheter. J Ultrasound Med 2018;37(9):2147–56.

32. Picone O, Benachi A, Mandelbrot L, et al. Thoracoamniotic shunting for fetal pleural effusions with hydrops. Am J Obstet Gynecol 2004;191(6):2047–50.

33. Mussat P, Dommergues M, Parat S, et al. Congenital chylothorax with hydrops: postnatal care and outcome folloing antenatal diagnosis. Acta Paediatr 1995;84(7):749–55.

34. White SB, Tutton SM, Rilling WS, et al. Percutaneous in utero thoracoamniotic shunt creation for fetal thoracic abnormalities leading to nonimmune hydrops. J Vasc Interv Radiol 2014;25(6):889–94.

35. Morris R, Malin G, Quinlan-Jones E, et al. The Percutaneous shunting in Lower Urinary Tract Obstruction (PLUTO) study and randomised controlled trial: evaluation of the effectiveness, cost-effectiveness and acceptability of percutaneous vesicoamniotic shunting for lower urinary tract obstruction. Health Technol Assess 2013;17(59):1–232.

36. Jeong BD, Won HS, Lee MY, et al. Perinatal outcomes of fetal pleural effusion following thoracoamniotic shunting. Prenat Diagn 2015;35(13):1365–70.

37. Petersen SG, Gibbons KS, Luks FI, Lewi L, Diement A, Hecher K, Dickinson JE, Stirnemann JJ, Vile Y, Devlieger R, Gardener G, Deprest JA.

38. Papanna R, Block-Abraham D, Mann LK, et al. Risk factors associated with preterm delivery after fetoscopic laser ablation for twin-twin transfusion syndrome. Ultrasound Obstet Gynecol 2014;433:48–53.

39. Malshe A, Snowise S, Mann LK, et al. Preterm delivery after fetoscopic laser surgery for twin-twin transfusion syndrome: etiology and risk factors. Ultrasound Obstet Gynecol 2017;49(5):612–6.
40. Ruegg L, Husler M, Krahenmann F, et al. Outcome after fetoscopic laser coagulation in twin-twin transfusion syndrome- is the survival rate of at least one child at 6 months of age dependent on the preoperative cervical length and preterm prelabor rupture of fetal membranes? J Matern Fetal Neonatal Med 2020;33(5): 852–60.
41. Papanna R, Molina S, Moise KY, et al. Chorioamnioplugging and the risk of preterm premature rupture of membranes after laser surgery in twin-twin transfusion syndrome. Ultrasound Obstet Gynecol 2010;35:337–43.
42. Habli M, Bombrys A, Lewis D, et al. Incidence of complications in twin-twin transfusion syndrome after selective fetoscopic laser photocoagulation: a single center experience. Am J Obstet Gynecol 2009;201(4):417.e1-7.
43. Hecher K, Lewi L, Gratacos E, et al. Twin reversed arterial perfusion: fetoscopic laser coagulation of placental anastomoses or the umbilical cord. Ultrasound Obstet Gynecol 2006;28:688–91.
44. Buyukkaya A, Tekbas G, Buyukkaya R. Twin Reversed Arterial Perfusion (TRAP) sequence; characteristic gray-scale and doppler ultrasonography findings. Iranian J Radiol 2015;12(3):e14979.
45. Paramasivam G, Wimalasundera R, Wiechec M, et al. Radiofrequency ablation for selective reduction in complex monochorionic pregnancies. BJOG 2010;117: 1294–8.
46. Moise KJ Jr, Johnson A, Moise KY, et al. Radiofrequency ablation for selective reduction in the complicated monochorionic gestation. Am J Obstet Gynecol 2008;198:198.e1-5.
47. Livingston JC, Lim FY, Polzin W, et al. Intrafetal radiofrequency ablation for twin reversed arterial perfusion (TRAP): a single center experience. Am J Obstet Gynecol 2007;197(4):399.e1-3.
48. Lee H, Wagner AJ, Sy E, et al. Efficacy of radiofrequency ablation for twin-reversed arterial perfusion sequence. Am J Obstet Gynecol 2007;196(5): 459.e1-4.
49. Lee H, Bebbington M, Crombleholm TM. The North American fetal therapy network registry data on outcomes of radiofrequency ablation for twin-reversed arterial perfusion sequence. Fetal Diagn Ther 2013;33:224–9.
50. Kohl T, Tchatcheva K, Merz W, et al. Percutaneous fetoscopic patch closure of human spina bifida aperta: advances in fetal surgical techniques may obviate the need for early postnatal neurosurgical intervention. Surg Endosc 2009; 23(4):890–5.
51. Kohl T, Tchatcheva K, Weinbach J, et al. Partial amniotic carbon dioxide insufflation (PACI) during minimally invasive fetoscopic surgery: early clinical experience in humans. Surg Endosc 2010;24(2):432–44.
52. Kohl T. Percutaneous minimally invasive fetoscopic surgery for spina bifida aperta. Part I: surgical technique and perioperative outcome. Ultrasound Obstet Gynecol 2014;44:515–24.
53. Pedreira DA, Zanon N, de Sá RA, et al. Fetoscopic single-layer repair of open spina bifida using a cellulose patch: preliminary clinical experience. J Matern Fetal Neonatal Med 2014;27:1613–9.
54. Kabagambe SK, Jensen GW, Chen YJ, et al. Fetal surgery for myelomeningocele: a systematic review and meta-anaylsis of outcomes in fetoscopic versus open repair. Fetal Diagn Ther 2018;43:161–74.

55. Belfort MA, Whitehead WE, Shamshirsaz AA, et al. Fetoscopic repair of meningomyelocele. Obstet Gynecol 2015;126:881–4.
56. Belfort MA, Whitehead WE, Shamshirsaz AA, et al. Fetoscopic open neural tube defect repair: development and refinement of a two-port, carbon dioxide insufflation technique. Obstet Gynecol 2017;129(4):734–43.
57. Graf K, Kohl T, Neubauer BA, et al. Percutaneous minimally invasive fetoscopic surgery for spina bifida aperta. Part III: neurosurgical intervention in the first postnatal year. Ultrasound Obstet Gynecol 2016;47:158–61.
58. Verbeek RJ, Heep A, Maurits NM, et al. Fetal endoscopic myelomeningocele closure preserved segmental neurological function. Dev Med Child Neurol 2012;54(1):15–22.
59. Sanz Cortes M, Davila I, Torres P, et al. Does fetoscopic or open repair for spina bifida affect fetal and postnatal growth? Ultrasound Obstet Gynecol 2019;53(3): 314–23.
60. Degenhardt J, Schurg R, Winarno A, et al. Percutaneous minimal-access fetoscopic surgery for spina bifida aperta. Part II: maternal management and outcome. Ultrasound Obstet Gynecol 2014;44(5):525–31.
61. Sola JE, Bronson SN, Cheung MC, et al. Survival disparities in newborns with congenital diaphragmatic hernia: a national perspective. J Pediatr Surg 2010; 45:1336–42.
62. Snoek KG, Greenough A, van Rosmalen J, et al. Congenital diaphragmatic hernia: 10-year evaluation of survival, extracorporeal membrane oxygenation, and foetoscopic endotracheal occlusion in four high-volume centres. Neonatology 2018;113:63–8.
63. Jani JC, Cordier AG, Martinovic J, et al. Antenatal ultrasound prediction of pulmonary hypoplasia in congenital diaphragmatic hernia: correlation with pathology. Ultrasound Obstet Gynecol 2011;38:344–9.
64. Deprest J, Gratacos E, Nicolaides KH. Fetoscopic tracheal occlusion (FETO) for severe congenital diaphragmatic hernia: evolution of a technique and preliminary results. Ultrasound Obstet Gynecol 2004;24(2):121–6.
65. Ruano R, Peiro JL, da Silva MM, et al. Early fetoscopic tracheal occlusion for extremely severe pulmonary hypoplasia in solated congenital diaphragmatic hernia: preliminary results. Ultrasound Obstet Gynecol 2013;42(1):70–6.
66. Jani JC, Nicolaides KH, Gratacos E, et al. Severe diaphragmatic hernia treated by fetal endoscopic tracheal occlusion. Ultrasound Obstet Gynecol 2009;34: 304–10.
67. Baschat AA, Rosner M, Millard SE, et al. Single-center outcome of fetoscopic tracheal balloon occlusion for severe congenital diaphragmatic hernia. Obstet Gynecol 2020;135(3):511–21.
68. Adzick NS, Thom EA, Spong CY, et al. A randomized trial of prenatal versus postnatal repair of myelomeningocele. N Engl J Med 2011;364:993–1004.
69. Sacco A, van der Veeken L, Bagshaw E, et al. Maternal complications following open and fetoscopic fetal surgery: a systematic review and meta-analysis. Prenat Diagn 2019;39(4):251–68.
70. Moron AF, Barbosa M, Milani H, et al. 771: short-term surgical and clinical outcomes with a novel method for open fetal surgery of myelomeningocele. Am J Obstet Gynecol 2015;212:S374.
71. Moron AF, Barbosa MM, Milani HJF, et al. Perinatal outcomes after open fetal surgery for myelomeningocele repair: a retrospective cohort study. BJOG 2018;125(10):1280–6.

72. Chang J, Tracy TF, Carr SR, et al. Port insertion and removal techniquies to minimize premature rupture of the membranes in endoscopic fetal surgery. J Pediatr Surg 2006;41(5):905–9.

73. Engels AC, Van Calster B, Richter J, et al. Collagen plug sealing of iatrogenic fetal membrane defects after fetoscopic surgery for congenital diaphragmatic hernia. Ultrasound Obstet Gynecol 2014;43:54–9.

74. Quintero RA, Romero R, Dzieczkowski J, et al. Sealing of ruptured amniotic membranes with intra-amniotic platelet-cryoprecipitate plug. Lancet 1996; 347(9008):1117.

75. Mann LK, Papanna R, Moise KJ, et al. Fetal membrane path and biomimetic adhesive coacervates as a sealant for fetoscopic defects. Acta Biomater 2012; 8(6):2160–5.

76. Kwak HM, Choi HJ, Cha HH, et al. Amniopatch treatment for spontaneous previable, preterm premature rupture of membranes associated or not with incompetent cervix. Fetal Diagn Ther 2013;33(1):47–54.

77. Deprest J, Emonds MP, Richter J, et al. Amniopatch for iatrogenic rupture of the fetal membranes. Prenat Diagn 2011;31(7):661–6.

78. Maged AM, Kamel HH, Sanad AS, et al. The value of amniopatch in pregnancies associated with spontaneous preterm premature rupture of fetal membranes: a randomized controlled trial. J Matern Fetal Neonatal Med 2019. https://doi.org/10.1080/14767058.2019.1605348. e1-7.

79. Chmait RH, Kontopoulos EV, Chon AH, et al. Amniopatch treatment of iatrogenic preterm premature rupture of membranes (iPPROM) after fetoscopic laser surgery for twin-twin transfusion syndrome. J Matern Fetal Neonatal Med 2017; 30(11):1349–54.

80. Simhan HN, Canavan TP. Preterm premature rupture of membranes: diagnosis, evaluation, and management strategies. BJOG 2005;112(1):32–7.

81. Friedman ML, McElin TW. Diagnosis of ruptured fetal membranes. Clinical study and review of the literature. Am J Obstet Gynecol 1969;104:544–50.

82. Bennett SL, Cullen JB, Sherer DM, et al. The ferning and nitrazine tests of amniotic fluid between 12 and 41 weeks gestation. Am J Perinatol 1993;10:101–4.

83. Adekola H, Gill N, Sakr S, et al. Outcomes following intra-amniotic instillation with indigo carmine to diagnose prelabor rupture of membranes in singleton pregnancies: a single center experience. J Matern Fetal Neonatal Med 2016; 29:544–9.

84. Beckmann MW, Wiegratz I, Dereser MM, et al. Diagnostik des Blasensprungs: Vergleich des vaginalen Nachweises von fetalem Fibronektin und der intraamnialen Injektion von Indigo Carmine. Geburtshilfe Frauenheilkd 1993;53:86.

85. Pakrashi T, Defranco EA. The relative proportion of preterm births complicated by premature rupture of membranes in multifetal gestations: a population-based study. Am J Perinatol 2013;30(1):69–74.

86. Mercer BM, Crocker LG, Pierce WF, et al. Clinical characteristics and outcome of twin gestation complicated by preterm premature rupture of membranes. Am J Obstet Gynecol 1993;168(5):1467–73.

87. Trentacoste SV, Jean-Pierre C, Baergen R, et al. Outcomes of preterm premature rupture of membranes in twin pregnancies. J Matern Fetal Neonatal Med 2008;21:555–7.

88. Myles TD, Espinoza R, Meyer W, et al. Preterm premature rupture of membranes: comparison between twin and singleton gestations. J Matern Fetal Med 1997;6:159–63.

89. Hsieh YY, Chang CC, Tsai HD, et al. Twin versus singleton pregnancy. Clinical characteristics and latency periods in preterm premature rupture of membranes. J Reprod Med 1999;44:616–20.
90. Jacquemyn Y, Noelmans L, Mahieu L, et al. Twin versus singleton pregnancy and preterm prelabour rupture of the membranes. Clin Exp Obstet Gynecol 2003;30:99–102.
91. Ural S, Deren O, Onderoglu L, et al. Does preterm premature rupture of membranes of one twin affect outcomes within twin gestations? Am J Obstet Gynecol 2006;195(6):S115.
92. Wagner P, Sonek J, Mayr S, et al. Outcome of dichorionic diamniotic twin pregnancies with spontaneous PPROM before 24 weeks' gestation. J Matern Fetal Med 2017;30(14):1750–4.
93. Wong LF, Holmgren CM, Silver RM, et al. Outcomes of expectantly managed pregnancies with multiple gestations and preterm premature rupture of membranes prior to 26 weeks. Am J Obstet Gynecol 2015;212(2):215.e1-9.
94. Committee on Practice Bulletins-Obstetrics. ACOG practice bulletin no. 188: prelabor rupture of membranes. Obstet Gynecol 2018;131(1):e1–14.
95. Kenyon SL, Taylor DJ, Tarnow-Mordi W, ORACLE Collaborative Group. Broad-spectrum antibiotics for preterm, prelabour rupture of fetal membranes: the ORACLE I randomised trial. Lancet 2001;357:979–88.
96. Ballabh P, Lo ES, Kumari J, et al. pharmacokinetics of betamethasone in twin and singleton pregnancy. Clin Pharmacol Ther 2002;71:39–45.
97. Blickstein I, Reichman B, Lusky A, et al. Plurality-dependent risk of severe intra ventricular hemorrhage among very low birth weight infants and antepartum corticosteroid treatment. Am J Obstet Gynecol 2006;194:1329–33.
98. Battista L, Winovitch KC, Rumney PJ, et al. A case-control comparison of the effectiveness of betamethasone to prevent neonatal morbidity and mortality in preterm twin and singleton pregnancies. Am J Perinatol 2008;25:449–53.
99. Doyle LW, Crowther CA, Middleton P, et al. Magnesium sulphate for women at risk of preterm birth for neuroprotection of the fetus. Cochrane Database Syst Rev 2009;(21):CD004661.
100. Bianco AT, Stone J, Lapinski R, et al. The clinical outcome of preterm premature rupture of membranes in twin versus singleton pregnancies. Am J Perinatol 1996;13(3):135–8.
101. Von Dadelszen P, Kives S, Delisle MF, et al. The association between early membrane rupture, latency, clinical chorioamnionitis, neonatal infection, and adverse perinatal outcomes in twin pregnancies complicated by preterm prelabour rupture of membranes. Twin Res 2003;6(4):257–62.

Neonatal and Childhood Outcomes Following Preterm Premature Rupture of Membranes

Lillian B. Boettcher, MD, Erin A.S. Clark, MD*

KEYWORDS

- Chorioamnionitis • Cerebral palsy • Fetal inflammatory response syndrome (FIRS)
- Intrauterine inflammation • Neurodevelopmental delay
- Neurodevelopmental outcomes • Preterm birth
- Preterm premature rupture of membranes (PPROM)

KEY POINTS

- Preterm premature rupture of membranes (PPROM) complicates approximately one-third of preterm births and is associated with significant, and unique, neonatal and childhood morbidity.
- Gestational age at membrane rupture and birth are the primary predictors of short-term and long-term outcomes for fetuses exposed to PPROM.
- Intrauterine inflammation/infection and oligohydramnios often accompanying PPROM may confer differential risks compared with other phenotypes of preterm birth.

INTRODUCTION

Preterm birth and its perinatal sequelae complicate approximately 10% of pregnancies in the United States.[1,2] Preterm premature rupture of membranes (PPROM) complicates approximately one-third of preterm births and is associated with significant, and unique, neonatal morbidity and mortality.[3,4] PPROM is almost uniformly associated with preterm birth and therefore complications related to prematurity explain much of the morbidity associated with this condition. The neonatal implications of chorioamniotic membrane rupture and subsequent preterm birth before 37 weeks' gestation are well established and may include periventricular leukomalacia (PVL), bronchopulmonary dysplasia (BPD), necrotizing enterocolitis (NEC), and retinopathy of prematurity (ROP). Broad implementation of antenatal risk reduction strategies,

Department of Obstetrics and Gynecology, University of Utah School of Medicine, Suite 2B200, 30 North 1900 East, Salt Lake City, UT 84132, USA
* Corresponding author.
E-mail address: erin.clark@hsc.utah.edu

Obstet Gynecol Clin N Am 47 (2020) 671–680
https://doi.org/10.1016/j.ogc.2020.09.001
0889-8545/20/© 2020 Elsevier Inc. All rights reserved.

such as maternal corticosteroids, and improvements in neonatal critical care have reduced these morbidities and improved survival in the modern medical era. Consequently, the longer-term sequelae of premature birth and exposure to the intrauterine environment of PPROM deserve dedicated study and discussion. This article reviews the mechanisms by which PPROM might uniquely confer neonatal morbidity, as well as updating the current understanding of the longer-term implications, focusing on neurologic outcomes, for children born after PPROM.

PATHOPHYSIOLOGY OF MORBIDITY

PPROM may simultaneously impose several disadvantageous conditions, including prematurity, intrauterine inflammation and infection, and oligohydramnios (**Fig. 1**). The risk factors within this unique environment may confer fetal and neonatal injury through a variety of pathways and mechanisms discussed here.

Prematurity

Most pregnancies complicated by PPROM deliver preterm and it is the magnitude of prematurity that inflicts a list of known and predictable adverse neonatal and childhood outcomes. A robust body of literature shows that gestational age at birth seems to be the strongest single predictor of morbidity and mortality in infants born after PPROM.[3] The PPROM event is followed by a period of latency, or duration of rupture before the onset of labor, ranging from hours to several weeks.[5] The latency period confers particular risks, including infection, placental abruption, and cord accident, but may also provide an opportunity to administer risk-reducing interventions before delivery, as discussed elsewhere in this issue. Because prematurity bestows most of the fetal and neonatal risk in PPROM, expectant management in the absence of contraindications remains the most critical risk reduction strategy.[3] The degree of prematurity and its direct and indirect consequences are primarily responsible for the wide spectrum of neonatal and childhood outcomes observed following PPROM.

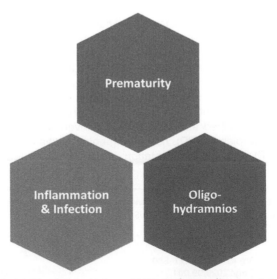

Fig. 1. The causal hat-trick of neonatal morbidity and mortality associated with PPROM.

Gestational age at delivery

Gestational age at delivery is the most important determinant of short-term neonatal outcomes following PPROM, superseding the risk factor of intra-amniotic infection.[6] Modern cohort studies that have compared infants of a similar gestational age following preterm birth from PPROM versus other causes have shown largely similar risk of mortality, repeat hospitalizations, and developmental outcomes.[7] In 7-year follow-up of the ORACLE I and II trials of antibiotics for women with PPROM and spontaneous labor with intact membranes, respectively, parent-reported functional impairment and educational performance were similar between infants, regardless of membrane status at trial enrollment.[8,9] Smaller single-center studies have suggested a higher risk of adverse neurodevelopmental outcomes with PPROM,[10–12] and whether differential risk is conferred by PPROM remains controversial and is discussed in more detail later. However, the preponderance of evidence strongly suggests that gestational age at birth, rather than the pathway to preterm birth, is the primary driver of short-term and long-term outcomes.

Gestational age at membrane rupture

Although gestational age at birth is most predictive of outcomes, gestational age at membrane rupture and associated latency remain critically important influences. When controlling for gestational age at delivery and other confounders, earlier gestational age at membrane rupture is significantly associated with neonatal death as well as neonatal and childhood morbidity.[13,14]

Periviable membrane rupture, addressed in more detail in a separate article in this series, deserves particular consideration because it is associated with the highest neonatal and childhood morbidity and mortality. Historically, outcomes in this situation have been very poor and counseling has emphasized a grim neonatal prognosis. However, more modern data suggest better outcomes than previously estimated. In the prospective EPIPAGE-2 (epidemiological study on small for gestational age children) cohort, which included 379 pregnancies with PPROM between 22 and 25 weeks, 52% of fetuses survived to discharge, 39% survived to discharge without severe morbidity, and 46% survived to 2 years without cerebral palsy (CP).[15] In a retrospective cohort study of 87 pregnancies with PPROM between 14 and 24 weeks, 23% of the infants survived to discharge, half of whom had normal neurodevelopmental outcome at 2 years of age.[16] In another retrospective cohort of 140 pregnancies with PPROM between 20 and 23 weeks, 49% survived to discharge, 53% survived to discharge without severe morbidity, and 77% of survivors had no demonstrable long-term morbidity at 18 to 21 months.[17] Keeping in mind the selection biases that accompany these studies, which largely report outcomes of pregnancies selected for expectant management, it is now clear that a nonnegligible proportion of children survive periviable membrane rupture without severe morbidity at the time of hospital discharge and at the time of later childhood evaluation. As such, counseling should attempt to convey the full spectrum of possible neonatal and childhood outcomes that are associated with periviable PPROM in pregnancies managed expectantly. Acknowledging regional differences in neonatal outcomes, this counseling should also attempt to incorporate local/institutional outcome data whenever possible.

Latency after rupture of membranes

Gestational age at the time of PPROM is inversely related to the subsequent length of latency. Latency after PPROM is variable and can range from hours to several weeks, with most women delivering within 1 week of presentation.[5] In an analysis of PPROM before 32 weeks in the era of antibiotics for pregnancy prolongation, the mean latency period was 9 days for PPROM occurring between 24 and 28 weeks, whereas at 29 weeks and beyond the latency period progressively shortened.[18] After membrane rupture occurs, the interval before onset of labor represents a period of susceptibility to the fetus as well as an opportunity to administer risk-reducing interventions. Consider that latency must meet a certain minimum duration to permit the risk reduction associated with antenatal interventions such as maternal corticosteroids and antibiotic prophylaxis, which are discussed in detail in other articles in this series.

Fetal and neonatal morbidity seems to vary according to the duration of latency, although inconsistently. In a prospective cohort study of PPROM cases between 24 and 34 weeks, 37% experienced a latency period shorter than 48 hours before onset of labor.[19] Before 30 weeks' gestation, a duration of rupture less than 48 hours was associated with higher infant mortality; pulmonary disease was determined to be the major cause of death. This effect was hypothesized to be mediated by differential exposure to antenatal corticosteroids. In contrast, a shorter latency period was associated with lower mortality after 30 weeks. In surviving infants, there were no neurologic implications associated with duration of latency at 2-year follow-up.

In a large retrospective study, Walker and colleagues[20] found that PPROM latency greater than or equal to 3 weeks was associated with increased mortality and decreased likelihood of survival without morbidity within all gestational age subgroups analyzed. In secondary analyses of the BEAM (Beneficial Effects of Antenatal Magnesium Sulfate) randomized controlled trial of magnesium sulfate, PPROM longer than 3 weeks was an independent risk factor for motor and mental delay, as shown by Bayley scores less than 70 at 2 years of age, but not CP.[21,22] These findings suggest that length of time exposed to the intrauterine environment of PPROM may be an independent predictor of neurodevelopmental delay.

Importantly, although these findings highlight that, at a given gestational age, prolonged latency may be a risk factor for adverse neurodevelopmental outcomes, it is important to remember that gestational age is the primary determinant of morbidity and mortality. Therefore, despite the possible adverse conditions imposed by the PPROM environment, prolongation of the latency period in appropriate candidates is the most critical modifiable factor to improve overall outcomes.

Birthweight

Consistent with several prior studies showing the association between intrauterine fetal growth restriction on childhood neurodevelopment,[23] small for gestational age (SGA) has been independently associated with an increased risk of adverse outcome in the setting of PPROM. In a secondary analysis of the BEAM trial of antenatal magnesium sulfate for preterm neuroprotection, Grace and colleagues[24] evaluated the independent impact of birthweight on composite adverse neonatal outcomes following PPROM. SGA infants were more likely to have major neonatal morbidity, including death, before hospital discharge. The mechanism by which SGA might contribute to these adverse outcomes is unclear, but placental disorder may be a unifying diagnosis.

Inflammation and Infection

The cause of PPROM is multifactorial and may include overt or subclinical intrauterine infection or inflammation.[4,25] Earlier gestational age at the time of PPROM is associated with higher incidence of coexisting infection.[26,27] Compared with other entries into preterm labor, neonatal sepsis occurs at a significantly higher rate in PPROM than induced or spontaneous preterm labor.[28]

Neurodevelopment

The neurodevelopmental sequelae of prematurity have been well described.[29] The inflammatory environment often associated with PPROM, in addition to the preterm delivery itself, may uniquely contribute to the risk for adverse neurodevelopmental outcomes.[30] PPROM is an independent risk factor for developing chorioamnionitis, a condition that in turn increases the risk of developing PVL and CP.[31–33] Causes of CP are numerous and multifactorial, and include perinatal hypoxia-ischemia, ischemic stroke, white matter disorders, congenital malformations, and intrauterine inflammation and infection.[34,35] Attention to inflammation as a key cause in adverse neurodevelopmental outcomes such as CP has increased over time, perhaps buoyed by an increase in molecular and cellular studies that permit a more nuanced understanding not appreciated with neuroimaging and clinical studies alone. As such, inflammation is now generally regarded as an essential component in the pathophysiology of fetal brain injury.[36] This notion that inflammation, and not simply preterm birth alone, is necessary to alter neuronal morphology has also been supported by murine models.[37]

Commonly observed in preterm infants exposed to inflammation, PVL describes the condition in which subcortical axonal white matter adjacent to the cerebral ventricles is damaged, leading to cell death and the development of cystic, fluid-filled spaces, a condition referred to as cystic PVL. Because critical motor tracts pass through this periventricular region, PVL is a strong independent risk factor for CP.[38] The most prominent risk factors identified for white matter injury are inflammatory conditions and cytokine exposure.[39] The fetal inflammatory response syndrome (FIRS) refers to the fetal innate immune response to intrauterine infection, marked by systemic increases in levels of inflammatory cytokines and chemokines, many of which have been identified in the pathophysiology of preterm birth and its sequelae.[40,41] Intrauterine infection/inflammation, prominent in PPROM, leads to release of proinflammatory cytokines into the fetal circulation. Levels of the cytokine interleukin (IL)-6 are increased in umbilical cord plasma in neonates who develop white matter injury and PVL; levels of the cytokines tumor necrosis factor-alpha (TNF-α), IL-6, and IL-1β are increased in amniotic fluid in fetuses that ultimately develop CP.[42]

The evidence for fetal brain injury occurring secondary to inflammation is especially pertinent to the PPROM story, because inflammatory processes may be present and in themselves may incite membrane rupture or develop subsequently. The resulting brain injury may manifest as CP and a spectrum of cognitive and behavioral disorders in children born after PPROM.

Lung development

Fetal exposure to inflammation also likely modifies fetal pulmonary immune cells and alters lung development.[43] Clinical observations consistently suggest that preterm infants exposed to inflammation, including ruptured membranes and histologic chorioamnionitis, are less likely to have respiratory distress syndrome (RDS).[44,45] The concept that fetal inflammation may induce lung maturation and increase responsiveness to maternal corticosteroids has been demonstrated in animal models.[43] In contrast, chorioamnionitis may increase the incidence of BPD in preterm infants.[44,46,47] Animal models suggest that fetal inflammatory exposures may modulate postnatal lung function and lung development.[43] In this way, the intrauterine inflammatory environment may affect the risk of short-term and long-term pulmonary morbidity in infants born preterm. This possibility may also explain why the diagnoses of RDS and BPD are not always correlated and predictable; they are not simply a reflection of gestational age but are a reflection of the unique characteristics of the intrauterine environment.

Other neonatal outcomes: necrotizing enterocolitis and retinopathy of prematurity
The inflammatory environment often associated with PPROM also has the potential to influence the risk of adverse outcomes in other organ systems. NEC has a multifactorial cause and primarily occurs in preterm infants. Gestational age, birthweight, and feeding method (bottle vs breastfeeding) are highly recognized risk factors.[48] Observational studies have also shown that chorioamnionitis and prolonged rupture of membranes, factors commonly associated with PPROM, are also strong risk factors.[49,50]

Recent data suggest that exposure to perinatal infection/inflammation might also be associated with increased risk of ROP. Although early gestational age, low birth weight, and oxygen supplementation after birth are perinatal risk factors consistently associated ROP, intrauterine infection/inflammation and the subsequent FIRS may increase sensitization to postnatal insults that lead to the development of ROP.[51–53]

Inflammation: molecular level
The picture of how the inflammatory pathophysiology inflicts fetal and neonatal damage is complex and incomplete. Further, the immune response may emanate from the maternal host and/or neonate. Funisitis is the histologic equivalent of the fetal inflammatory response, whereas chorioamnionitis represents a maternal inflammatory response. In chorioamnionitis, neutrophils infiltrate from the maternal decidua.[54] In murine models mimicking neonatal exposure to intrauterine inflammation, exposure to even low-dose lipopolysaccharide induces significant increases in messenger RNA expression of TNF-α, IL-1β, and cyclooxygenase-2.[55]

IL-17A, a proinflammatory cytokine produced by lymphocytes of the innate immune system and residing in barrier tissue, is necessary for clearing extracellular pathogens. IL-17A is a key instigator of innate immunity and a mediator of FIRS.[36,41] In murine models, IL-17A is robustly produced in the setting of inflammatory sepsis stimulated by IL-18.[56] The specific mechanism of IL-17A–induced cortical brain injury may include impaired migration of immature postmitotic neurons from the ventricular zone to the neocortex.[36] In addition, IL-17A triggers neutrophil recruitment in cerebral blood vessels, which may lead to microvascular obstruction and further exacerbation of neurologic injury through propagation of the inflammatory response and production of reactive oxygen species.[36] Increased IL-18 levels are associated with production of proinflammatory molecules, such as interferon-gamma, TNF-α, and IL-1, which have been implicated in preterm labor and neonatal brain injury.[40] Further, systemic activation of toll-like receptor-4 (TLR-4) has also been implicated in central nervous system white matter damage.[40,57] This finding was recently shown in an animal study of the intrauterine environment; the absence of TLR-4 prevented fetal brain injury in the setting of intrauterine inflammation.[58]

Clinically, molecular markers of fetal inflammation, including IL-1β, IL-6, IL-8, and TNF-α, have been associated with adverse neurologic outcomes following PPROM, independent of gestational age at birth or cranial ultrasonography findings.[59] Understanding of the association between the fetal inflammatory response, the molecular markers at play, and resultant perinatal brain injuries seen in pregnancies complicated by preterm birth and PPROM is continuing to evolve.

Oligohydramnios

When PPROM occurs, it is often associated with severely reduced levels of amniotic fluid. Prolonged oligohydramnios can result in fetal musculoskeletal and soft tissue deformations, some of which may resolve after birth.[3] More importantly, and particularly when PPROM occurs in the midtrimester, it may lead to pulmonary hypoplasia and hypoxic respiratory failure in the neonate. Inadequate circulating amniotic fluid, especially during the critical midtrimester, may result in decreased potential airway and air space distention in the fetus. This condition may lead to lower lung weights and volumes, impaired parenchymal maturation, reduced airspaces, reduced elastin, decreased cell size, and decreased chest wall compliance.[60,61] Clinically, this translates to severe respiratory morbidity and high neonatal mortality, particularly when PPROM occurs before 24 weeks' gestation, when critical early lung development is still in process.[62] Both retrospective and prospective cohort data suggest that survival and developmental outcomes are adversely affected by persistent oligohydramnios compared with normal amniotic fluid volume after PPROM.[63,64]

SUMMARY

Preterm birth resulting from PPROM remains a critical public health problem and is associated with significant perinatal morbidity and mortality. Although prematurity and its associated complications explain much of the morbidity and mortality associated with PPROM, it is prudent to remember the unique maternal and fetal environment that accompanies this condition. Understanding that environment, and its molecular underpinnings, is necessary to understand the causal mechanisms of the neonatal and childhood outcomes that are observed, which may be disparate from other pathways to preterm birth. Ultimately, a better understanding of these mechanisms, and the underlying genetic and environmental interactions, is key to developing new antenatal and postnatal risk reduction strategies. Funding research that extends follow-up into childhood will be critical in order to implement novel strategies that improve long-term morbidity following PPROM.

DISCLOSURE

The authors have nothing to disclose.

REFERENCES

1. Martin JA, Hamilton BE, Osterman MJK, et al. Births: Final Data for 2018. Natl Vital Stat Rep 2019;68(13):1–47.
2. Matthews TJ, MacDorman MF, Thoma ME. Infant Mortality Statistics From the 2013 Period Linked Birth/Infant Death Data Set. Natl Vital Stat Rep 2015; 64(9):1–30.
3. Prelabor Rupture of Membranes: ACOG Practice Bulletin Summary, Number 217. Obstet Gynecol 2020;135(3):739–43.
4. Goldenberg RL, Culhane JF, Iams JD, et al. Epidemiology and causes of preterm birth. Lancet 2008;371(9606):75–84.
5. Mercer BM. Preterm premature rupture of the membranes. Obstet Gynecol 2003; 101(1):178–93.
6. Rodríguez-Trujillo A, Cobo T, Vives I, et al. Gestational age is more important for short-term neonatal outcome than microbial invasion of the amniotic cavity or intra-amniotic inflammation in preterm prelabor rupture of membranes. Acta Obstet Gynecol Scand 2016;95(8):926–33.
7. Roberts CL, Wagland P, Torvaldsen S, et al. Childhood outcomes following preterm prelabor rupture of the membranes (PPROM): a population-based record linkage cohort study. J Perinatology 2017;37(11):1230–5.
8. Kenyon S, Pike K, Jones DR, et al. Childhood outcomes after prescription of antibiotics to pregnant women with preterm rupture of the membranes: 7-year follow-up of the ORACLE I trial. Lancet 2008;372(9646):1310–8.

9. Kenyon S, Pike K, Jones DR, et al. Childhood outcomes after prescription of antibiotics to pregnant women with spontaneous preterm labour: 7-year follow-up of the ORACLE II trial. Lancet 2008;372(9646):1319–27.

10. Patkai J, Schmitz T, Anselem O, et al. Neonatal and two-year outcomes after rupture of membranes before 25 weeks of gestation. Eur J Obstet Gynecol Reprod Biol 2013;166(2):145–50.

11. Spinillo A, Capuzzo E, Stronati M, et al. Effect of preterm premature rupture of membranes on neurodevelopmental outcome: follow up at two years of age. Br J Obstet Gynaecol 1995;102(11):882–7.

12. Kieffer A, Pinto Cardoso G, Thill C, et al. Outcome at Two Years of Very Preterm Infants Born after Rupture of Membranes before Viability. PLoS One 2016;11(11): e0166130.

13. Manuck TA, Varner MW. Neonatal and early childhood outcomes following early vs later preterm premature rupture of membranes. Am J Obstet Gynecol 2014; 211(3):308.e1-6.

14. Accordino F, Consonni S, Fedeli T, et al. Risk factors for cerebral palsy in PPROM and preterm delivery with intact membranes (.). J Matern Fetal Neonatal Med 2016;29(23):3854–9.

15. Lorthe E, Torchin H, Delorme P, et al. Preterm premature rupture of membranes at 22-25 weeks' gestation: perinatal and 2-year outcomes within a national population-based study (EPIPAGE-2). Am J Obstet Gynecol 2018;219(3): 298.e1--14.

16. Pristauz G, Bauer M, Maurer-Fellbaum U, et al. Neonatal outcome and two-year follow-up after expectant management of second trimester rupture of membranes. Int J Gynecol Obstet 2008;101(3):264–8.

17. Kibel M, Asztalos E, Barrett J, et al. Outcomes of Pregnancies Complicated by Preterm Premature Rupture of Membranes Between 20 and 24 Weeks of Gestation. Obstet Gynecol 2016;128(2):313–20.

18. Peaceman AM, Lai Y, Rouse DJ, et al. Length of latency with preterm premature rupture of membranes before 32 weeks' gestation. Am J Perinatol 2015;32(1):57–62.

19. Pasquier JC, Bujold E, Rabilloud M, et al. Effect of latency period after premature rupture of membranes on 2 years infant mortality (DOMINOS study). Eur J Obstet Gynecol Reprod Biol 2007;135(1):21–7.

20. Walker MW, Picklesimer AH, Clark RH, et al. Impact of duration of rupture of membranes on outcomes of premature infants. J Perinatol 2014;34(9):669–72.

21. Drassinower D, Friedman AM, Obican SG, et al. Prolonged latency of preterm prelabour rupture of membranes and neurodevelopmental outcomes: a secondary analysis. BJOG 2016;123(10):1629–35.

22. Drassinower D, Friedman AM, Običan SG, et al. Prolonged latency of preterm premature rupture of membranes and risk of cerebral palsy. J Matern Fetal Neonatal Med 2016;29(17):2748–52.

23. Levine TA, Grunau RE, McAuliffe FM, et al. Early childhood neurodevelopment after intrauterine growth restriction: a systematic review. Pediatrics 2015;135(1): 126–41.

24. Grace MR, Dotters-Katz S, Varner MW, et al. Birthweight Extremes and Neonatal and Childhood Outcomes after Preterm Premature Rupture of Membranes. Am J Perinatol 2016;33(12):1138–44.

25. Goldenberg RL, Hauth JC, Andrews WW. Intrauterine infection and preterm delivery. N Engl J Med 2000;342(20):1500–7.

26. Garite TJ, Freeman RK. Chorioamnionitis in the preterm gestation. Obstet Gynecol 1982;59(5):539–45.

27. Ramsey PS, Lieman JM, Brumfield CG, et al. Chorioamnionitis increases neonatal morbidity in pregnancies complicated by preterm premature rupture of membranes. Am J Obstet Gynecol 2005;192(4):1162–6.

28. Pinto S, Malheiro MF, Vaz A, et al. Neonatal outcome in preterm deliveries before 34-week gestation – the influence of the mechanism of labor onset. J Matern Fetal Neonatal Med 2019;32(21):3655–61.

29. Saigal S, Doyle LW. An overview of mortality and sequelae of preterm birth from infancy to adulthood. Lancet 2008;371(9608):261–9.

30. Clark EA, Varner M. Impact of preterm PROM and its complications on long-term infant outcomes. Clin Obstet Gynecol 2011;54(2):358–69.

31. Yoon BH, Park CW, Chaiworapongsa T. Intrauterine infection and the development of cerebral palsy. BJOG 2003;110(Suppl 20):124–7.

32. Wu YW, Colford JM Jr. Chorioamnionitis as a risk factor for cerebral palsy: A meta-analysis. JAMA 2000;284(11):1417–24.

33. Yoon BH, Romero R, Park JS, et al. Fetal exposure to an intra-amniotic inflammation and the development of cerebral palsy at the age of three years. Am J Obstet Gynecol 2000;182(3):675–81.

34. Nelson KB. Causative factors in cerebral palsy. Clin Obstet Gynecol 2008;51(4): 749–62.

35. van Lieshout P, Candundo H, Martino R, et al. Onset factors in cerebral palsy: A systematic review. Neurotoxicology 2017;61:47–53.

36. Lawrence SM, Wynn JL. Chorioamnionitis, IL-17A, and fetal origins of neurologic disease. Am J Reprod Immunol 2018;79(5):e12803.

37. Burd I, Bentz AI, Chai J, et al. Inflammation-induced preterm birth alters neuronal morphology in the mouse fetal brain. J Neurosci Res 2010;88(9):1872–81.

38. Deng W, Pleasure J, Pleasure D. Progress in periventricular leukomalacia. Arch Neurol 2008;65(10):1291–5.

39. Leviton A, Paneth N, Reuss ML, et al. Maternal infection, fetal inflammatory response, and brain damage in very low birth weight infants. Developmental Epidemiology Network Investigators. Pediatr Res 1999;46(5):566–75.

40. Hagberg H, Mallard C, Jacobsson B. Role of cytokines in preterm labour and brain injury. BJOG 2005;112(Suppl 1):16–8.

41. Gotsch F, Romero R, Kusanovic JP, et al. The fetal inflammatory response syndrome. Clin Obstet Gynecol 2007;50(3):652–83.

42. Yoon BH, Jun JK, Romero R, et al. Amniotic fluid inflammatory cytokines (interleukin-6, interleukin-1beta, and tumor necrosis factor-alpha), neonatal brain white matter lesions, and cerebral palsy. Am J Obstet Gynecol 1997;177(1):19–26.

43. Kramer BW, Kallapur S, Newnham J, et al. Prenatal inflammation and lung development. Semin Fetal Neonatal Med 2009;14(1):2–7.

44. Watterberg KL, Demers LM, Scott SM, et al. Chorioamnionitis and early lung inflammation in infants in whom bronchopulmonary dysplasia develops. Pediatrics 1996;97(2):210–5.

45. Andrews WW, Goldenberg RL, Faye-Petersen O, et al. The Alabama Preterm Birth study: polymorphonuclear and mononuclear cell placental infiltrations, other markers of inflammation, and outcomes in 23- to 32-week preterm newborn infants. Am J Obstet Gynecol 2006;195(3):803–8.

46. Van Marter LJ, Dammann O, Allred EN, et al. Chorioamnionitis, mechanical ventilation, and postnatal sepsis as modulators of chronic lung disease in preterm infants. J Pediatr 2002;140(2):171–6.

47. Viscardi RM, Muhumuza CK, Rodriguez A, et al. Inflammatory markers in intrauterine and fetal blood and cerebrospinal fluid compartments are associated

with adverse pulmonary and neurologic outcomes in preterm infants. Pediatr Res 2004;55(6):1009–17.

48. Rose AT, Patel RM. A critical analysis of risk factors for necrotizing enterocolitis. Semin Fetal Neonatal Med 2018;23(6):374–9.

49. Been JV, Lievense S, Zimmermann LJ, et al. Chorioamnionitis as a risk factor for necrotizing enterocolitis: a systematic review and meta-analysis. J Pediatr 2013; 162(2):236–42.e2.

50. Ahle M, Drott P, Elfvin A, et al. Maternal, fetal and perinatal factors associated with necrotizing enterocolitis in Sweden. A national case-control study. PLoS One 2018;13(3):e0194352.

51. Lee J, Dammann O. Perinatal infection, inflammation, and retinopathy of prematurity. Semin Fetal Neonatal Med 2012;17(1):26–9.

52. Chen M, Citil A, McCabe F, et al. Infection, oxygen, and immaturity: interacting risk factors for retinopathy of prematurity. Neonatology 2011;99(2):125–32.

53. Chen ML, Allred EN, Hecht JL, et al. Placenta microbiology and histology and the risk for severe retinopathy of prematurity. Invest Ophthalmol Vis Sci 2011;52(10): 7052–8.

54. Kim CJ, Romero R, Chaemsaithong P, et al. Acute chorioamnionitis and funisitis: definition, pathologic features, and clinical significance. Am J Obstet Gynecol 2015;213(4 Suppl):S29–52.

55. Elovitz MA, Brown AG, Breen K, et al. Intrauterine inflammation, insufficient to induce parturition, still evokes fetal and neonatal brain injury. Int J Dev Neurosci 2011;29(6):663–71.

56. Wynn JL, Wilson CS, Hawiger J, et al. Targeting IL-17A attenuates neonatal sepsis mortality induced by IL-18. Proc Natl Acad Sci U S A 2016;113(19): E2627–35.

57. Breen K, Brown A, Burd I, et al. TLR-4-dependent and -independent mechanisms of fetal brain injury in the setting of preterm birth. Reprod Sci 2012;19(8):839–50.

58. Tulina NM, Brown AG, Barila GO, et al. The Absence of TLR4 Prevents Fetal Brain Injury in the Setting of Intrauterine Inflammation. Reprod Sci 2019;26(8):1082–93.

59. Armstrong-Wells J, Donnelly M, Post MD, et al. Inflammatory predictors of neurologic disability after preterm premature rupture of membranes. Am J Obstet Gynecol 2015;212(2):212.e1-9.

60. de Waal K, Kluckow M. Prolonged rupture of membranes and pulmonary hypoplasia in very preterm infants: pathophysiology and guided treatment. J Pediatr 2015;166(5):1113–20.

61. Najrana T, Ramos LM, Abu Eid R, et al. Oligohydramnios compromises lung cells size and interferes with epithelial-endothelial development. Pediatr Pulmonol 2017;52(6):746–56.

62. Waters TP, Mercer BM. The management of preterm premature rupture of the membranes near the limit of fetal viability. Am J Obstet Gynecol 2009;201(3): 230–40.

63. Lee JY, Ahn TG, Jun JK. Short-Term and Long-Term Postnatal Outcomes of Expectant Management After Previable Preterm Premature Rupture of Membranes With and Without Persistent Oligohydramnios. Obstet Gynecol 2015; 126(5):947–53.

64. Pergialiotis V, Bellos I, Fanaki M, et al. The impact of residual oligohydramnios following preterm premature rupture of membranes on adverse pregnancy outcomes: a meta-analysis. Am J Obstet Gynecol 2020;222(6):628–30.

UNITED STATES POSTAL SERVICE ® Statement of Ownership, Management, and Circulation (All Periodicals Publications Except Requester Publications)

1. Publication Title	2. Publication Number	3. Filing Date
OBSTETRICS AND GYNECOLOGY CLINICS OF NORTH AMERICA	000 – 276	9/18/2020

4. Issue Frequency	5. Number of Issues Published Annually	6. Annual Subscription Price
MAR, JUN, SEP, DEC	4	$325.00

7. Complete Mailing Address of Known Office of Publication (Not printer) (Street, city, county, state, and ZIP+4®)

ELSEVIER INC.
230 Park Avenue, Suite 800
New York, NY 10169

Contact Person
Malathi Samayan

Telephone (Include area code)
91-44-4299-4507

8. Complete Mailing Address of Headquarters or General Business Office of Publisher (Not printer)

ELSEVIER INC.
230 Park, Avenue, Suite 800
New York, NY 10169

9. Full Names and Complete Mailing Addresses of Publisher, Editor, and Managing Editor (Do not leave blank)

Publisher (Name and complete mailing address)

Editor (Name and complete mailing address)

KERRY HOLLAND, ELSEVIER INC.
1600 JOHN F KENNEDY BLVD. SUITE 1800
PHILADELPHIA, PA 19103-2899

Managing Editor (Name and complete mailing address)

PATRICK MANLEY, ELSEVIER INC.
1600 JOHN F KENNEDY BLVD. SUITE 1800
PHILADELPHIA, PA 19103-2899

10. Owner (Do not leave blank. If the publication is owned by a corporation, give the name and address of the corporation immediately followed by the names and addresses of all stockholders owning or holding 1 percent or more of the total amount of stock. If not owned by a corporation, give the names and addresses of the individual owners. If owned by a partnership or other unincorporated firm, give its name and address as well as those of each individual owner. If the publication is published by a nonprofit organization, give its name and address.)

Full Name	Complete Mailing Address
WHOLLY OWNED SUBSIDIARY OF REED/ELSEVIER, US HOLDINGS	1600 JOHN F KENNEDY BLVD. SUITE 1800 PHILADELPHIA, PA 19103-2899

11. Known Bondholders, Mortgagees, and Other Security Holders Owning or Holding 1 Percent or More of Total Amount of Bonds, Mortgages, or Other Securities. If none, check box ☑ None

Full Name	Complete Mailing Address
N/A	

12. Tax Status (For completion by nonprofit organizations authorized to mail at nonprofit rates) (Check one)
The purpose, function, and nonprofit status of this organization and the exempt status for federal income tax purposes:
☑ Has Not Changed During Preceding 12 Months
☐ Has Changed During Preceding 12 Months (Publisher must submit explanation of change with this statement)

PS Form 3526, July 2014 (Page 1 of 4 (see instructions page 4)) PSN: 7530-01-000-9931   PRIVACY NOTICE: See our privacy policy on www.usps.com.

13. Publication Title	14. Issue Date for Circulation Data Below
OBSTETRICS AND GYNECOLOGY CLINICS OF NORTH AMERICA	JUNE 2020

15. Extent and Nature of Circulation		Average No. Copies Each Issue During Preceding 12 Months	No. Copies of Single Issue Published Nearest to Filing Date
a. Total Number of Copies (Net press run)		215	172
b. Paid Circulation (By Mail and Outside the Mail)	(1) Mailed Outside-County Paid Subscriptions Stated on PS Form 3541 (Include paid distribution above nominal rate, advertiser's proof copies, and exchange copies)	54	45
	(2) Mailed In-County Paid Subscriptions Stated on PS Form 3541 (Include paid distribution above nominal rate, advertiser's proof copies, and exchange copies)	0	0
	(3) Paid Distribution Outside the Mails Including Sales Through Dealers and Carriers, Street Vendors, Counter Sales, and Other Paid Distribution Outside USPS®	109	91
	(4) Paid Distribution by Other Classes of Mail Through the USPS (e.g. First-Class Mail®)	0	0
c. Total Paid Distribution (Sum of 15b (1), (2), (3), and (4))		163	136
d. Free or Nominal Rate Distribution (By Mail and Outside the Mail)	(1) Free or Nominal Rate Outside-County Copies included on PS Form 3541	34	17
	(2) Free or Nominal Rate In-County Copies Included on PS Form 3541	0	0
	(3) Free or Nominal Rate Copies Mailed at Other Classes Through the USPS (e.g. First-Class Mail)	0	0
	(4) Free or Nominal Rate Distribution Outside the Mail (Carriers or other means)	34	17
e. Total Free or Nominal Rate Distribution (Sum of 15d (1), (2), (3) and (4))		34	17
f. Total Distribution (Sum of 15c and 15e)		197	153
g. Copies not Distributed (See Instructions to Publishers #4 (page #3))		18	19
h. Total (Sum of 15f and g)		215	172
i. Percent Paid (15c divided by 15f times 100)		82.74%	88.89%

* If you are claiming electronic copies, go to line 16 on page 3. If you are not claiming electronic copies, skip to line 17 on page 3.

16. Electronic Copy Circulation	Average No. Copies Each Issue During Preceding 12 Months	No. Copies of Single Issue Published Nearest to Filing Date
a. Paid Electronic Copies ▶		
b. Total Paid Print Copies (Line 15c) + Paid Electronic Copies (Line 16a) ▶		
c. Total Print Distribution (Line 15f) + Paid Electronic Copies (Line 16a) ▶		
d. Percent Paid (Both Print & Electronic Copies) (16b divided by 16c × 100) ▶		

☑ I certify that 50% of all my distributed copies (electronic and print) are paid above a nominal price.

17. Publication of Statement of Ownership

☑ If the publication is a general publication, publication of this statement is required. Will be printed in the DECEMBER 2020 issue of this publication.   ☐ Publication not required.

18. Signature and Title of Editor, Publisher, Business Manager, or Owner

Malathi Samayan   Date 9/18/2020

Malathi Samayan - Distribution Controller

I certify that all information furnished on this form is true and complete. I understand that anyone who furnishes false or misleading information on this form or who omits material or information requested on the form may be subject to criminal sanctions (including fines and imprisonment) and/or civil sanctions (including civil penalties).

PS Form 3526, July 2014 (Page 2 of 4)   PRIVACY NOTICE: See our privacy policy on www.usps.com.

Printed and bound by CPI Group (UK) Ltd, Croydon, CR0 4YY

03/10/2024

01040405-0015